# AN
# ASPIRIN
# A DAY

## *About the Author*

Dr Keith Souter graduated in Medicine from the University of Dundee in 1976 and worked as a family doctor in Wakefield for almost thirty years. The general practice at which he worked contributed statistics to the Royal College of General Practitioners Weekly Returns Service and was part of the Medical Research Council's General Practice Research Framework. As such, Dr Souter was involved in several national trials, including one of the major studies on aspirin.

He has been a medical columnist for twenty-eight years and is a medical journalist, although he still practises medicine. He is a prolific author and has written over twenty books, including eleven novels and several health books, such as *Doctors' Latin*, *Coping with Rheumatism and Arthritis*, *50 Things That You Can Do to Manage Back Pain*, and *Now You're Talking*.

He is a Fellow of the Royal College of General Practitioners, and a member of the Medical Journalists' Association, the Society of Authors, the Crime Writers' Association and International Thriller Writers. He is happily married and has three grown-up children and a granddaughter.

# AN ASPIRIN A DAY

**The Wonder Drug That Could Save *YOUR* Life**

### Dr Keith Souter

FOREWORD BY PROFESSOR TOM MEADE FRS

MICHAEL O'MARA BOOKS LIMITED

First published in Great Britain in 2011 by
Michael O'Mara Books Limited
9 Lion Yard
Tremadoc Road
London SW4 7NQ

Copyright © Michael O'Mara Books Limited 2011

All rights reserved. No part of this publication may be reproduced, stored in a retrieval system, or transmitted by any means, without the prior permission in writing of the publisher, nor be otherwise circulated in any form of binding or cover other than that in which it is published and without a similar condition including this condition being imposed on the subsequent purchaser.

A CIP catalogue record for this book is available from the British Library.

Papers used by Michael O'Mara Books Limited are natural, recyclable products made from wood grown in sustainable forests. The manufacturing processes conform to the environmental regulations of the country of origin.

**Disclaimer**: The information contained in this book is correct to the best of the author and publisher's knowledge and contains the latest research at the time of publication. It is *not* an alternative to seeking personalized medical advice. **Before anyone commits to taking aspirin on a daily basis, they should have a consultation with their own doctor. Aspirin is *not* suitable for everyone.** Both the author and the publisher disclaim any responsibility from any medical consequences that may occur. Please also note: neither the author nor the publisher has any relationship whatsoever with any pharmaceutical company.

ISBN: 978-1-84317-632-9

1 3 5 7 9 10 8 6 4 2

Designed and typeset by E-Type

Illustrations on pages 45, 69 and 74 by David Woodroffe

Printed and bound in Great Britain by CPI Cox & Wyman, Reading, RG1 8EX

www.mombooks.com

# Contents

*Author's Acknowledgements* — 6
*Foreword* by Professor Tom Meade FRS — 7
*A Note on How to Use This Book* — 10

Introduction — 12
1 Aspirin: The Highlights — 14
2 Aspirin: The Wonder Drug? — 19
3 The History of Aspirin — 31
4 How Aspirin Works — 45
5 Pain, Fever and Inflammation — 55
6 The Heart and Circulation — 67
7 Strokes — 94
8 Arteries, Veins and Aspirin in Pregnancy — 104
9 Aspirin and Dementia — 117
10 Cancer: A Short Overview — 126
11 Colorectal Cancer — 145
12 Cancer of the Lung — 153
13 Breast Cancer — 157
14 Cancer of the Prostate — 161
15 Aspirin in Diabetes — 166
16 Depression — 171
17 The Skin — 181
18 Unusual Uses of Aspirin — 184
19 Aspirin: Side Effects and Precautions — 196
Conclusion: Aspirin Reflections — 207

*Glossary of Terms* — 209
*References* — 214
*Index* — 221

# Author's Acknowledgements

I would like to thank Professor Tom Meade FRS for taking the time to write the Foreword to this book, which highlights the need for continuing research into this simple yet very important drug.

I would also like to thank Kate Moore, commissioning editor at Michael O'Mara, both for commissioning the book and for her deft touch with the editorial pen. Thank you too to David Woodroffe for his illustrations.

As always, thanks to Isabel Atherton, my agent at Creative Authors, who started my journey through the history and research on aspirin that has become this book.

And finally, thanks to my wife Rachel for her support during the many long hours when I was working away in my study.

# Foreword

*by Professor Tom Meade FRS*

Only forty years ago – quite a short time as these things go – aspirin was really only used for pain relief and for lowering the temperature during fever. True, laboratory studies in the late 1960s had shown that aspirin inhibits platelet clumping or aggregability. However, it was not until 1974 that the first trial of aspirin in secondary prevention, i.e. in men who had already had a heart attack (myocardial infarction), was published in the *British Medical Journal* from the MRC (Medical Research Council) Epidemiology Unit in South Wales.[1] It was a small, underpowered trial and not much notice was paid to it at the time. But the same group published another trial soon after, and gradually other investigators carried out their own secondary prevention trials. It was the large international ISIS-2 trial[2] published in *The Lancet* in 1988 that made the greatest impact. The trial was a factorial evaluation of two drugs, aspirin 160mg (enteric coated) and streptokinase 1.5 MU infusion, soon after the onset of myocardial infarction. Each agent on its own lowered vascular mortality within the next 35 days by about 25 per cent, while the rate was reduced by just over 40 per cent in those allocated to both agents. A survey soon after the trial showed that the trial had had an unusually swift and quite remarkable effect on clinical practice, so that the combination of aspirin and streptokinase became virtually routine treatment in those with recent onset myocardial infarction.

By 2002 the Antithrombotic Trialists' Collaboration[3], having gathered the individual patient data from all the secondary prevention trials that had been carried out, left no doubt that aspirin reduced serious vascular events by a quarter, vascular mortality by a sixth, non-fatal myocardial infarction by a third and non-fatal stroke by a quarter. It was clear that the benefit of aspirin greatly outweighed the risk of serious bleeding, so that aspirin in those who had had cardiac or vascular episodes at other sites became standard treatment for both short- and long-term secondary prevention.

The value of aspirin in secondary prevention raised the obvious question – would it be useful in primary prevention as well, that is, preventing first episodes in those who had not previously experienced any? So far, six primary prevention trials have reported and their combined experience was written up in *The Lancet* in 2009.[4] As with secondary prevention, aspirin resulted in a large reduction, by about 20 per cent, in non-fatal heart attacks. But, unlike the secondary prevention results, there was no clear benefit in terms of either stroke or death from fatal heart attacks. Vascular mortality was not reduced. Compared with secondary prevention, these results are puzzling. On the one hand, it is reasonably argued that there is a continuum of severity of pathological changes in coronary arteries, so that it is hard to imagine a point at which aspirin confers no benefit but then becomes beneficial. On the other hand, it shouldn't be assumed that the pathological background and the responsiveness to aspirin are necessarily the same in those previously affected or unaffected by clinical events.

Whatever the explanation, one clear contrast with secondary prevention has emerged. While the benefit attributable to aspirin in those who have previously had vascular events clearly outweighs the risk of serious bleeding, the same can't be said in the context of primary prevention, where benefit only begins to outweigh hazard in those at high risk of events. This should make doctors recommend aspirin only cautiously to patients who haven't had heart or stroke problems. Furthermore, it may be that those who self-medicate with aspirin through over-the-counter purchases are potentially doing themselves more harm than good.

Very recently, aspirin has sprung another surprise – the likelihood that after it has been taken for about five years, it reduces mortality rates from several cancers by substantial amounts, particularly those of the gastrointestinal tract.[5]

Aspirin therefore benefits the two major causes of death – cardiovascular disease and cancer. The findings on cancer need to be taken into account along with those on vascular disease, tipping the previous balance more towards benefit than harm. In primary and secondary prevention of vascular disease and taking account of its effect on cancer mortality as well, it seems that an aspirin dose of 75mg daily is as effective as higher doses, with almost certainly less risk of serious bleeding.

Aspirin is cheap and, provided it is used with care, it is relatively free of serious hazards, though the possibility of serious gastrointestinal or cerebral bleeding should not to be overlooked. Whoever you are – medical professional or lay reader – what single medication would you choose if you could only have one from now on? Might it be aspirin?

Drawing on his years in general practice and on his writing skills, Dr Keith Souter is ideally placed to answer these and other questions about aspirin.

*Professor Tom Meade FRS*

# A NOTE ON HOW TO USE THIS BOOK

It is not the intention of the author or of the publisher that readers should regard this book as a substitute for a medical opinion from their own doctor. Indeed, its aim is to lay before the interested reader information about the history, science and research that has been done on aspirin over the years, presenting the results so that readers can learn more for themselves about this extraordinary drug.

Low dose aspirin has undoubted potential benefits for many people, provided that there are clear indications as to why it could help them reduce their risk of various conditions. On the other hand, aspirin does have a number of potential side effects, some of which are very serious.

**No one should just start taking regular aspirin.** Before anyone commits to taking this drug on a daily basis, they should have a consultation with their own doctor in order to assess their level of risk for the various conditions discussed in this book. This should be balanced against the risk of any of the side effects that are possible. If you have risk factors for several conditions, e.g. both cardiovascular disease and some types of cancer, then your decision may be fairly simple.

The question of whether or not someone who is currently well, with a seemingly low risk of cardiovascular disease or cancer, should take aspirin as a *primary* preventive is more difficult. If you are simply considering it as a preventive against one group of diseases, then you may be swayed against taking it because of the risk of side effects. If you are considering its potential against both groups, then you may consider that the benefits far outweigh the risks. A look at the research that has been done on aspirin in these different areas may help you to make that decision.

In order to compile this book, I have read a vast number of research papers on aspirin. At this point I feel I should add that the interpretation of those trials and papers is mine alone. I have aimed to be accurate and present findings in as clear a manner as possible, in order to give a balanced view about the drug.

Essentially, the whole reason for this book is to help both the reader and his or her doctor come to an informed decision about whether they should consider using aspirin as a preventive agent against cardiovascular disease, cancer, Alzheimer's disease, or other conditions – an aspirin a day.

*Dr Keith Souter*

## A note on the glossary

I have at all times aimed to make this book accessible to everybody who has an interest in learning more about aspirin and its potential for health, regardless of medical knowledge and training.

To that end, I explain any medical terms used in the book when they are first introduced, and I have also compiled a glossary of terms as a one-stop reference point, in case you encounter an unfamiliar phrase later in the book.

I suspect some readers may consult only those chapters relevant to their own health concerns, and would therefore like to point readers in the direction of the glossary of terms located at the back of this book on page 209, which I hope will be of use.

# INTRODUCTION

I have always had a healthy respect for aspirin. This predates my entrance to medical school by a dozen years and my qualification as a doctor by eighteen years. Quite simply, aspirin transformed my father's life.

According to my mother, our family doctor told her that aspirin actually saved his life. In retrospect, I do not think that his life was actually at risk at that time, although he undoubtedly had a case of rheumatic fever, some of the complications of which can be extremely serious.

I vividly remember the treatment he was given with large doses of aspirin, the daily visits by the silver-haired doctor, and the sense of relief in the family when the sick room, from which I was excluded, became instead a visiting room, where I could see my father recover and convalesce.

In a sense, aspirin was one of the reasons that I decided to become a doctor myself.

When I was at medical school, aspirin was going through one of its periodic falls from favour. New drugs had been developed that had bypassed it in popularity, so that it had become regarded as little more than a household remedy.

Then some spectacular research revealed that aspirin was anything but a remedy to be despised and disparaged. It had beneficial effects that no one had realized before when it was taken in low dose, *just an aspirin a day.*

Over the last thirty-five years, I have been fascinated to see the continued rehabilitation of aspirin. In low dose, it proved to be effective in reducing the risk of having heart attacks and strokes, and also seemed to reduce the risk of some types of cancer. Gradually, the number of conditions that it reduces the risk of having has increased. Most recently, a huge study covering 25,000 patients (from Oxford University and several other centres) has shown that a small daily dose of aspirin could substantially reduce the overall cancer death rate when it has been taken regularly for a period of five years or more.

Before I became a medical journalist, I was the partner responsible for research and for coordinating data collection within my general practice, which was one of the contributing practices on the Medical Research Council's GP Research Framework. I was delighted when one of the trials we worked on showed a positive result in terms of aspirin's ability to reduce the risk of having a first heart attack. I am proud to have contributed, albeit in a very minor way as a mere data collector, to a trial that has had an impact upon clinical practice.

Since then, more and more research has been published about aspirin, the way it seems to work and the range of conditions that it may have a role in preventing. Most recently, a large trial suggests that it may substantially reduce the risk of *many* cancers.

Truly it seems that aspirin has come of age as 'the wonder drug'.

# ASPIRIN: THE HIGHLIGHTS

This book, in its entirety, offers a comprehensive and detailed analysis of aspirin, describing how it could help you with a range of medical conditions and providing an in-depth examination of the many ground-breaking studies into aspirin's role as a preventative drug.

However, this chapter simply presents the stark highlights of the drug's impact, so you can see – at a glance – the extraordinary results for yourself.

## Aspirin: the results

Aspirin has been proven to help with a range of medical conditions, including, but not limited to, heart attacks, strokes, cancer and dementia. Some of the results are quite astounding – and so here are the highlights. Scientific studies have drawn the following key conclusions.

## Heart attacks and strokes

- Aspirin is proven to help people who have already had a heart attack. In such patients, taking a low dose aspirin on

## ASPIRIN: THE HIGHLIGHTS

a daily basis reduces the risk of having another heart attack or a stroke by **at least one third**.
- Aspirin has also been shown to be effective at reducing the risk of a *first* heart attack in those patients at *high* risk of having a heart attack or stroke. Some studies reduced the risk of such events by **as much as 44 per cent**.
- When treating a heart attack, the death rate was reduced by **42 per cent** in patients who received a dual treatment of aspirin and streptokinase.

> While there is evidence of the benefit of taking aspirin for those people who are at *high* risk of having a heart attack or a stroke, the same evidence is not there for people at *low* risk who have *no* evidence of disease. While there may be a slight reduction in the risk of major events for such low-risk patients, this would have to be balanced against the risk of having a major bleed, one of the potential side effects of aspirin. The risks of having a bleed are discussed on page 198.

- If a patient has suffered a non-haemorrhagic stroke, the Royal College of Physicians recommends patients should be prescribed 50–300mg of aspirin daily **indefinitely**, as a preventative measure against further events.
- Patients who have had a mini-stroke should take aspirin. Studies have shown that taking aspirin reduces the odds of suffering another stroke by **15 per cent**.
- According to the National Institute for Health and Clinical Excellence (NICE) recommendations, patients with the commonest type of irregular heartbeat, called atrial fibrillation, who are classified at low or moderate risk of a stroke,

should be given aspirin in a daily dose of 75–300mg in order to prevent strokes and heart attacks.

## Cancer

- A small daily dose of aspirin has been proven to reduce the overall cancer death rate by **at least one fifth**.
- Aspirin needs to be taken for at least 5 years before an effect is seen in a reduction of the risk of cancer. After 5 years of taking aspirin, the death rate for all cancers fell by **34 per cent**.
- The longer the usage, the greater the reduction in risk: 20–25 years of usage gives the best protection. After that, there may be more risk of bleeds.
- The peak time to start to reap the benefit seems to be when patients are in their late forties and fifties.
- There is no difference in aspirin dose in this preventive role – 75mg seems sufficient to produce the effect.

### Specific types of cancer

- After 5 years of taking aspirin, the death rate for gastrointestinal cancers fell by **54 per cent**.
- Long-term use of aspirin is associated with a **30–50 per cent** reduction in the incidence of the polyps (tumours) which may lead to colorectal cancer, actual cancer of the colon and rectum, and death related to this disease. One study in particular showed that aspirin reduced the risk of proximal colon cancer (cancer nearest the small intestine, rather than near the rectum) by **70 per cent**.
- Aspirin reduced deaths due to primary brain tumours during the first 10 years of follow-up.
- The risk for prostate cancers fell after 15 years of aspirin usage.

Death rates dropped after 20 years of aspirin use:

- By **10 per cent** for prostate cancer.
- By **30 per cent** for lung cancer (but mainly for the adenocarcinoma type – defined on page 140 – which is more common in non-smokers).
- By **40 per cent** for colorectal cancer.
- By **60 per cent** for oesophageal cancer (of adenocarcinoma type).

### More research needed

- In one observational study into aspirin and patients with *existing* breast cancer, aspirin use was associated with a decreased risk for spread of cancer by **43–60 per cent**, and a **64–71 per cent** reduction in the risk for breast cancer-related death. While this study is promising, there is not yet enough research to suggest that well women should put themselves at risk of having an aspirin-related bleed in order to reduce their risk of breast cancer.
- The effect of aspirin on stomach, pancreatic and brain cancers is hard to determine at present, since insufficient numbers have been seen in studies to do a clear statistical analysis.
- Similarly, in the major studies, there have been too few women in the trials to determine the effects of aspirin on breast cancer or gynaecological cancers.

## Dementia

- Aspirin has been shown to reduce the risk of developing Alzheimer's disease by **23 per cent**.
- Studies have indicated that long-term use of aspirin may reduce the incidence of Alzheimer's disease, provided that the use has started well before the onset of dementia.

- The longer aspirin has been used, the greater the reduction in risk. For any benefit it seems that aspirin has to be taken long term, probably for at least 5 years.

## Can you take aspirin?

While aspirin is a drug that most people can take, to others it could be fatal.

You should NEVER take aspirin if you:

- Have a history of stomach ulceration
- Have a history of asthma
- Have had a haemorrhagic stroke
- Have any blood disorder or inherited condition such as Osler-Weber-Rendu disease (also known as hereditary haemorrhagic telangiectasia), which could predispose you to bleeding
- Have had an allergic reaction to aspirin at any time in your life
- Have a history of salicylate allergy
- Are under sixteen years old
- Are breastfeeding
- Are pregnant (unless prescribed aspirin by a doctor for a specific illness)
- Are trying to conceive
- Are on drugs like anticoagulants, or other drugs which could interact with aspirin to increase the risk of a bleed

Chapter 19 discusses these restrictions and the side effects of aspirin, so readers can make an informed choice about whether or not to take it.

These results are but the tip of a very large iceberg of aspirin studies. To understand the impact of the drug – and whether or not it is right for you – I would urge you now to read on, for more detail on this 'wonder drug' ... and how it could help to save *your* life.

# ASPIRIN: THE WONDER DRUG?

In the modern world we are used to superlatives. Whereas once there were models and film stars, now there are supermodels and megastars. Is the term a 'wonder drug' just another example of modern society's desire to show that everything is getting better?

In days gone by, people hoped that they would find a magical cure-all, a panacea for all ills. In fact, the word 'panacea' comes from the name of one of the goddesses who was quoted in the original Hippocratic Oath, the vow all doctors take when they enter the medical profession.

> *I swear by Apollo the physician, and Asclepias and Hygieia and Panacea and all the gods and goddesses of the pantheon ...*
>
> Thus began the original Hippocratic Oath, as first formulated by Hippocrates, the father of medicine, in Greece in the fifth century BC. Asclepius was the first god of medicine. Hygieia, the goddess of sanitation, and Panacea, the goddess of all cures, were his daughters.

## Can a wonder drug exist?

For a drug to be considered a panacea, it would have to work for everything, and that simply is not possible. The human body is so complex that a simple chemical, or even a cocktail of chemicals, could never affect all of the many processes that go on in a living cell. To imagine that a drug could deal with all of the many pathological processes that result in illness is therefore sheer fantasy.

An ideal drug, on the other hand, would not necessarily have to be a panacea. It would not have to deal with all ailments, but it would have to work *ideally* in certain conditions and circumstances.

For example, an ideal antibiotic would be one that treated all infections and produced no side effects. Similarly, an ideal painkiller would only alleviate pain. An ideal anti-cancer drug would kill cancerous cells, yet have no effect on the surrounding normal and healthy tissues.

Unfortunately, no drug fits the bill of maximum benefit and zero side effects.

## Enter aspirin

Aspirin is the most widely used drug in the world. About 35 metric tonnes are produced and consumed annually, which is enough to produce 100 billion tablets every year. It is readily available in most countries and can be bought over the counter in chemists, supermarkets, corner shops and even at the cash desks of garages.

It was taken to the Antarctic by Captain Robert Falcon Scott, to the top of Mount Everest by Edmund Hillary and to the Moon by the Apollo astronauts.

Aspirin is one of the most effective and versatile drugs that we know of, and every general practitioner will probably carry some in his bag, since it is known to be a life-saver after a heart attack.

The incredible thing is that, in one form or another, people have been using herbs or drugs containing aspirin-like substances for a range of conditions since the days of antiquity. The fact that these early medicines clearly worked led doctors and chemists to attempt to discover what the active ingredient was. We shall follow the convoluted history of aspirin in the next chapter.

## Chemical make-up

The actual chemical in aspirin is called acetylsalicylic acid. It is a surprisingly simple molecule with the formula $C_9H_8O_4$. The science of aspirin is crucial to our understanding of how this wonder drug exerts its many effects, so we shall consider the known science in chapter 4.

It was the first of the group of drugs that became known as the Non-Steroidal Anti-Inflammatory Drugs, or NSAIDs.

## Different forms of aspirin

Aspirin is usually taken in tablet form.

### Standard tablets

Available in 300mg or low dose 75mg

- They can be taken with or without food, although with food seems less likely to result in any gastric upsets. Taking a little milk or a glass of water also seems to help.

### Dispersible tablets

Available in 300mg or low dose 75mg

- They are dissolved or dispersed in a little water. Some people find these easier than having to swallow. A dispersed drug will also be less likely to erode the lining of the stomach, which a tablet lying directly in contact with the lining theoretically could do.

### Enteric-coated aspirin

Available in 300mg or 75mg

- These are given to people with sensitive stomachs. The theory is that the enteric coat will prevent the aspirin being dissolved in the stomach, but once it gets into the small intestine, it will be dissolved and absorbed. This will help reduce gastric irritation to an extent, but gastric side effects *are* still possible.

### Suppositories

Available in 300mg and 150mg

- As these are absorbed through the rectal mucosa, rather than the stomach, one would think that gastric side effects would be removed. However, gastric side effects are still possible.

## Aspirin – a drug full of paradoxes

The truth is that aspirin has always been a bit of a paradox. For most of the twentieth century, aspirin was considered one of the most successful painkilling and anti-rheumatic drugs available to doctors, yet many people seem reluctant to use it.

Sometimes this is due to reported side effects. Some patients found that they were unable to take aspirin because it caused gastric irritation, heartburn, stomach ulcers or seemed to promote minor bleeding disorders. As a consequence, many doctors became biased against aspirin because of its potential to cause such side effects – yet as this book will show, such side effects tend to be limited among patients and are certainly not as widespread as anti-aspirin propaganda would have you believe.

For others, the fact that aspirin is so readily available without the need of a doctor's prescription (although it is also obtainable on the NHS with a doctor's prescription) has tended to make people regard it as little more than a household remedy. In fact, more and more research is demonstrating that these small, white, unassuming tablets are veritable life-savers.

Perhaps most importantly, although its effectiveness as a painkiller and drug that can reduce fevers and inflammation has never been in doubt, aspirin's cheapness works strangely against it.

Psychologists tell us that people are liable to believe that a cheap drug is going to be of less value and benefit than a more expensive and more attractive tablet or capsule. This is fascinating, since there are considerable amounts of money to be made from the sale of different painkilling drugs. The pharmaceutical industry is highly competitive and potentially very lucrative. The fact that aspirin is cheap and therefore perceived by consumers to offer less benefit is of demonstrable financial value to the pharmaceutical industry, enabling them to promote alternative drugs – at higher cost to the consumer.

## Cheap as chips

So why is aspirin so cheap in some countries? Well, the reason is tied into the first global conflict of the twentieth century.

The name 'Aspirin' was originally patented by the German pharmaceutical company Bayer in 1899. Consequently, during the First World War, the Allies had difficulty in obtaining aspirin, so an alternative method of manufacture was devised, as we shall read about in chapter 3.

After the war, Germany was forced to make reparations. Part of this reparation meant that Bayer lost its registered trademark in France, England, the USA and Russia. Other companies could now make aspirin in these countries – and so the price of the drug dropped due to competition in the market.

## What's in a name?

Today, 'aspirin' is a generic word in Australia, France, India, Ireland, New Zealand, Pakistan, Jamaica, the Philippines, South Africa, the United Kingdom and the United States. This means that other pharmaceutical companies can prepare the drug under the name of aspirin. This makes it a cheap purchase in these countries.

However, Bayer still holds the trademark in about 80 countries around the world, including Germany, Switzerland, Canada and Mexico, where only *they* can market it as Aspirin. They use a capital A in their branding, but this is merely aesthetic: in countries where the trademark is held, no one else can use the name aspirin, with or without a capital letter. A generic drug in these countries can only be sold as acetylsalicylic acid, which doesn't sound quite so user-friendly. The trademarking also means that aspirin cannot be sold below a certain price, as Bayer alone determines this.

*Note:* For the purposes of this book, the generic version of 'aspirin' used in the UK, France and the USA will be used throughout, unless the Bayer-owned trademarked drug is referred to.

> ### THE MIRACLES OF ST ASPIRINIUS
>
> The selection of a suitable commercial name for acetylsalicylic acid was apparently no easy matter. There are two theories as to its origin, of which this may be the more fanciful. It is said that the drug was named after St Aspirinius, an early Neapolitan bishop, who reportedly became the patron saint of headaches.

## Aspirin vs paracetamol

There is not a great deal of money to be made from the sale of generic drugs such as aspirin. It is patented drugs, i.e. drugs that can be sold by only one company, that are the real money-spinners, since the company with the monopoly can set the price as high as the market will stand.

Consequently, for pharmaceutical companies there is a financial drive to promote patented drugs over generic drugs like aspirin – such as the various branded paracetamol-containing drugs that aspirin is often confused with.

Aspirin and paracetamol are very different drugs, although they are both effective painkillers and efficient at reducing fevers.

- Aspirin has significant anti-inflammatory effect, while paracetamol has little. Crucially, it is this anti-inflammatory effect that seems to give aspirin its great usefulness across a whole range of areas.
- On the other hand, paracetamol has a less irritant effect on the gastrointestinal system (but see the PAIN study on page 197 in chapter 19 on Side Effects and Precautions:

some paracetamol users do report gastrointestinal problems).

## Aspirin in practice

Over the years, aspirin has shown itself to be an amazingly effective drug. Indeed, while it undoubtedly has side effects that almost preclude its use by some people, its versatility is proving quite staggering.

It is important, however, to consider it as a drug that has two quite different areas in which it can be applied.

### As an actual treatment

Up until the 1970s it was known that aspirin was a drug that was effective as an:

- Analgesic (painkiller)
- Anti-pyretic (reduces fever)
- Anti-inflammatory (reduces inflammation)

These beneficial effects made it an effective agent in many conditions including rheumatism and arthritis, menstrual pain, minor aches and pains, and in the symptomatic treatment of various feverish illnesses.

It was a major drug in the treatment of the specific and very important condition of rheumatic fever, before the advent of antibiotics. It was also one of the most effective drugs against gout, although the high doses needed tended to produce gastric side effects.

For all of these conditions it is prescribed in a standard dose as a tablet containing 300mg.

## As a preventative drug

In the 1970s, aspirin was found to be effective in preventing platelets, a particular type of blood cell, from sticking together. By stopping this from happening, it prevents one of the first stages in blood clotting. Blood clots can be dangerous, leading to heart attacks and strokes, among other conditions, so this discovery was of major significance.

At first standard doses were prescribed, but research showed that low doses of 75–150mg daily were all that was needed to have a positive, preventative effect.

Over the last two decades, more and more research has revealed that low dose aspirin has a significant part to play in the prevention of various serious and potentially life-threatening illnesses.

* In the 1980s, a series of research studies demonstrated that aspirin was effective in reducing the risk of a second heart attack in people who had previously had one, or who had unstable angina.
* Other studies followed and showed that it also had a role in preventing a first heart attack in people who were at risk of heart disease. At the same time, it was demonstrated to be effective in reducing the risk of having certain types of strokes.
* Other research suggested that aspirin had a marked effect on reducing the risk of a whole variety of conditions, including Alzheimer's disease, depression, and various cancers. It was widely thought to have a role in reducing the risk of complications in diabetes.
* Towards the end of 2010, a major review was published based on research from Oxford University and other centres, covering over 25,000 patients. This found that a small daily dose of aspirin could reduce the overall cancer death rate by at least one fifth.

# The therapeutic uses of aspirin

## In full dose – as a treatment

Mild to moderate pain conditions
Headache
Migraine
Osteoarthritis
Rheumatoid arthritis
Psoriatic arthropathy
Other inflammatory rheumatic conditions
Pericarditis (inflammation of the sac that surrounds the heart)
Rheumatic fever (in high doses)
Kawasaki disease (see glossary)
Immediate treatment after a heart attack
Feverish colds and respiratory infections

## Low dose aspirin a day – as a preventive

Clotting disorders
Thrombo-phlebitis★
Deep-vein thrombosis★
Pulmonary embolism★
Atrial fibrillation
Coronary artery disease
Stroke prevention
Alzheimer's disease
Diabetes – to prevent complications★★
Retinal vein thrombosis
Retinopathy (when there is damage to the retina of the eye)
Nephropathy (when there is kidney damage)
Cataracts

# ASPIRIN: THE WONDER DRUG?

Cancers – several types, including:
* Colon
* Rectum
* Oesophagus
* Pancreas
* Breast
* Prostate
* Brain
* Lung

---

\* Although current medical opinion is that it is *not* indicated (shown to be effective) for these three conditions, as we shall see in chapter 8.

\*\* Though not currently indicated, *unless* there is evidence of pre-existing cardiovascular disease.

## Side effects of aspirin

As explained at the start of this chapter, no drug is in practice an ideal drug – and even the 'wonder drug' aspirin has side effects, as set out below.

### The most common

* Irritation of the stomach and intestines
* Indigestion and heartburn
* Nausea

To put this in proportion, about 6 per cent of people will experience some form of indigestion.

### Less common, but important

* Asthma induction, and spasms of the airways in the lungs (known as bronchospasm)
* Stomach ulceration

- Bleeding from the stomach
- Bruising
- Allergy – from the mildest, affecting the skin to produce nettle rash, to the severest, an anaphylactic reaction. Only about 0.5 per cent of patients experience an allergic reaction
- Haemorrhagic stroke
- Reye's syndrome (which affects children under sixteen years of age)

## In over-dosage

- Tinnitus (noises in the ears, most commonly ringing)
- Hyperglycaemia (rise in blood sugar levels)
- Increased body temperature
- Metabolic upsets (namely alterations in the acid-base balance in the body)

### CHAPTER SUMMARY

In conclusion, by virtue of its known ability to treat so many conditions when taken at a full dose, and to reduce the risk of death from the world's two major causes of death – heart disease and cancer – when taken at a small daily dose, in my opinion aspirin *can* legitimately claim to be that fabled beast: a wonder drug.

# THE HISTORY OF ASPIRIN

3

As mentioned in chapter 2, acetylsalicylic acid was first patented as the drug Aspirin in 1899. Technically, the history of aspirin starts from that time, yet that is only one milestone on a long winding trail that stretches back into the mists of time.

## The plant connection

The natural world holds the key to the origins of aspirin. Plants such as willow are rich in compounds called salicylates. These compounds give willow and other herbs their healing properties: a benefit that was discovered in the days of antiquity. It took almost five millennia before scientists extracted those compounds and developed aspirin as we know it today, but in its basest form it has been used as a medicine for millennia.

## The search begins with willow

Trying to trace the origins of aspirin is rather like asking a detective to pick up various clues and bits of evidence in order to build up a picture of a case.

It is entirely appropriate, therefore, to learn that Agatha Christie, the most celebrated detective writer of all time, met her future husband Max Mallowan when he was an assistant archaeologist working on an excavation at the ancient Sumerian city of Ur, located in modern-day southern Iraq – for this site holds the first clue in our quest to chart the history of the drug.

### The first clue – the ancient Sumerian clay tablet

One of the major finds at Ur was a clay tablet dating from about 3,000 BC, with cuneiform writing on it. Referred to as Ur III, this was a medical text from the Third Dynasty of Ur. It mentions several remedies, including salicylate-containing plants like myrtle and willow bark.

### The Ebers papyrus[1] – ancient Egypt

The next piece of evidence comes from ancient Egypt. In 1862, Edwin Smith, a young amateur Egyptologist and adventurer, purchased two papyri in Luxor. It is unclear from whom he bought them, but it is said that they had been found between the legs of a mummy in the El-Assasif area of the Theban necropolis on the other side of the Nile from Luxor.

Both of these papyri dated to about 1,534 BC, but were thought to be copies of far older texts. One became known as the Edwin Smith papyrus and is the oldest known surgical text in the world.

The other eventually fell into the hands of the German Egyptologist Georg Ebers in 1872. It is a medical text outlining the state of Egyptian knowledge about medicine and treatments of a wide range of conditions. Among the 160-odd remedies featured, the writers recorded the use of both willow, which they called *tjeret*, and myrtle, which they called *khet-des*, as well as cucumber, which they called *shespet*. All three of these are rich in salicylates.

> ### WHAT ARE SALICYLATES?
>
> Most plants contain some salicylates, but some are extremely rich in them. Plant physiologists have discovered that these act as plant hormones, which help a plant to flower and grow, but they also form one of the main defences that a plant may have against insects and other creatures. They are toxic to the intestines of insects and they are antiseptic against soil bacteria.
>
> Salicylates are what chemists later extracted from plants to create aspirin. These early uses of plants rich in salicylates – such as willow, myrtle and cucumber – are therefore the earliest uses of what came to be aspirin, albeit in a base form. The evidence shows that 'aspirin' has had a medical use for millennia.

## Hippocratic medicine

Hippocrates (*c.*460–380 BC) was an ancient Greek physician, commonly regarded as the 'father of medicine'. He was the first physician to reject superstition and demonic possession as a cause for illness, instead proposing that illness was due to an imbalance of various humors or vital fluids. This was the dominant medical theory until the Renaissance.

In his extensive writings, known collectively as the *Corpus Hippocraticum*, he advocated the use of a brew of willow leaves to control the pain of childbirth and to dispel fevers.

> ## THE DOCTRINE OF SIGNATURES
>
> The Doctrine of Signatures is an archaic theory which held that useful medicinal plants had special markings or clues that indicated their helpfulness in particular diseases.
>
> The willow – which grows in damp places where fevers and rheumatic problems are common – was known as a 'shiver tree', and indeed assisted with those shivers caused by fever. The use of willow in medicine is therefore an excellent example of the Doctrine of Signatures in practice.
>
> Although the Doctrine of Signatures seems naive to us today, it did appear to yield some effective treatments, of which willow – the natural origin of aspirin the wonder drug – is just one.

### Roman medicine and black cumin seeds

Pedanius Dioscorides of Anazarbus (AD 4–90) was a Greek physician born in Asia Minor in the Roman Empire. He wrote a five-volume book in Greek about the preparation, properties and testing of drugs, which was translated into Latin as *De materia medica*. It became the standard text on drugs for sixteen centuries.

He advocated the use of black cumin seeds for headaches and toothache, and wrote about the many useful properties of willow. Both are rich in salicylates.

### Roman medicine and willow leaves

Aulus Cornelius Celsus (25 BC–AD 50) was a Roman encyclopaedist, although thought not to have been a doctor. His book *de Medicina* is the only surviving text of a much larger encyclopaedia. It is a prime source on diet, medicine and surgery.

In this book, Celsus describes the four cardinal signs of inflammation as follows – *calor* (warmth), *dolor* (pain), *tumor* (swelling) and *rubor* (heat). He also advised using an extract of willow leaves to ease all of these. He can be regarded as being the first person to describe inflammation and to use willow specifically for its anti-inflammatory properties.

## Galen and the cooling ability of cucumber

Claudius Galenus of Pergamum (AD 131–201) was a famous second-century physician. He taught that cucumber was a 'cooling fruit', and advised that it be included in making up a Galenical medicine, the name for one of his formulations.

This is another example of the Doctrine of Signatures, the cucumber's 'signature' being that it was grown in hot conditions, yet when cut open it is always cooler inside (try it yourself and see). Thus it was used to cool temperatures, and when rubbed on parts of the body, it would cool and reduce inflammation. (Again, these effects are due to the salicylates that it contains). These properties are the origin of the phrase 'as cool as a cucumber'!

## Early medicine in the Americas

For centuries before the arrival of Christopher Columbus on the American continent, native American tribes had been using infusions of the bark and leaves of white willow to treat painful conditions and fevers. The Aztecs and Mayans of South America also independently discovered and used willow.

## Willow meets science

Though use of willow became firmly established as something of a 'folk remedy' through the centuries, its benefits (and, crucially, the reasons behind them) had yet to be explored by the scientific community by the time of the seventeenth century.

As it happened, malaria held the key to unlocking the secrets of its success for scientists. This disease – and treatments for it – had preoccupied doctors for millennia, with Hippocrates writing on it in the fifth century BC, when he called it 'swamp fever'.

In the mid-seventeenth century, powdered Peruvian Bark – known as chinchona – was extolled for its properties in the treatment of fevers. The problem was that Peruvian Bark was expensive. An alternative was required. Who knew that the search for one would ultimately result in the creation of aspirin?

### The Reverend Stone

A chance discovery by the Reverend Edward Stone (1702–68) in 1763, that powdered willow bark tasted like quinine, led him to use it as a substitute for chinchona bark.

To his delight and amazement, it seemed to have a range of activity beyond that of chinchona's ability to reduce fevers. Most significantly, it also had pain-relieving qualities. Crucially for the scientific community, he wrote about his discovery in a letter to the Royal Society, who published it in their *Philosophical Transactions* in 1763.

> *I treated five and forty of my parishioners who were suffering from various agues [fevers] with increasing doses of powdered willow bark ... and almost all of them rapidly improved.*

Significantly, Reverend Stone referred to the Doctrine of Signatures as being the reason that he was drawn to test willow bark. Although he does not say so, it is likely that he had been aware that willow preparations had been used in local folk medicine.

## The scientists' search

The Reverend Edward Stone was typical of the leisured professional man during the Age of Enlightenment. As a Church of England rector, he had sufficient security to indulge his interests in medicine, philosophy and astronomy. His fortunate discovery of willow bark opened up a whole new search. Just what was the wonder ingredient in the bark of an English shiver tree? The scientists now got to work.

> In 1828, Professor Johann Buchner at Munich University extracted a tiny amount of a bitter-tasting crystalline substance, which he called *salicin*. This was the active agent in willow.

> In 1830, a young French chemist, Henri Leroux, improved the process and was able to extract a larger and purer amount of salicin from willow bark.

> In 1838, the Italian chemist Rafaele Piria succeeded in splitting salicin into a sugar and an aromatic compound called salicylaldehyde. He was then able, by another chemical process, to convert that into a purer preparation, which he called *salicylic acid*.

**AN ASPIRIN A DAY**

Throughout the mid-eighteenth century, doctors prescribed salicin and salicylic acid with good results for many painful conditions, including arthritis, gout, rheumatic fever and typhoid fever.

Unfortunately, they also found that many people suffered from significant bleeding problems, gastric irritation and stomach ulceration. There was a need to find a less troublesome treatment.

---

In 1853, a French chemist, Charles Frederic Gerhardt, managed to 'buffer' salicylic acid with sodium and acetyl chloride to produce a chemical called *acetylsalicylic acid* (aka aspirin as we know it today). It was a major breakthrough, although Gerhardt did not realize it at the time. He gave up further work on it.

⬇

In 1859, Professor Adolph Kolbe synthesized salicylic acid from carbolic acid. The Kolbe-Schmitt synthesis eventually became the first step in the industrial manufacture of aspirin.

⬇

In 1870, Professor von Nencki of Basle demonstrated that salicin was converted into salicylic acid in the body. It would therefore make sense to give salicylic acid as a drug rather than the cruder salicin: saving the body the trouble of the conversion means the drug can get to work faster and with greater precision.

## The major breakthrough

In 1897, the German chemist Felix Hoffman, who was working for the pharmaceutical company Bayer, rediscovered Gerhardt's formula while he was looking for a way to produce a form of salicylic acid that would not produce stomach irritation. There was a personal motivation behind this: his father had found salicylic acid effective, but also found the gastric side effects too hard to cope with.

Using the herb meadowsweet as the source for salicylic acid, Hoffman gave his father various modified forms of salicylic acid in a type of clinical trial that would be ethically unacceptable today. Eventually, he managed to produce acetylsalicylic acid (aspirin) by using a different chemical process. The result was a form of acetylsalicylic acid that his father found worked extremely well.

By 1898, Hoffman was ready to launch his new drug. However, his immediate boss at Bayer, Heinrich Dreser, dismissed the new drug's market potential, since he suspected

### HEROIC EFFORTS

Felix Hoffman produced the drug known as heroin by accident, after attempting to create codeine from an opium poppy. It was given its name after the German *heroisch*, meaning 'heroic', which was the way that it made one feel. It was marketed as a non-addictive alternative to morphine for the treatment of pain, as well as a children's cough medicine.

Just as with Aspirin, the trademark was lost after the First World War. It is now illegal in most countries, although it is still prescribed and used in medicine as the strong painkiller, diamorphine.

that the drug would have 'an enfeebling effect' upon the heart – though the real reason apparently was that Bayer was about to market another of Hoffman's drugs, heroin.

Had it not been for Arthur Eichengrun, who was in charge of new drug development, the new drug might not have been released. As it was, he pressed for it and the drug was prepared for launch.

## Aspirin makes its debut

In 1899, Bayer patented the method of preparation of aspirin and obtained the trademark for it as Aspirin. I have already mentioned the more fanciful theory as to the origin of the name: that it was named after St Aspirinius, the patron saint of headaches. The more likely version is that it was a composite name derived from 'A' for *acetyl*; 'spir' for *Spiraea ulmaria* (meadowsweet) and 'in' … well, simply because that was a common ending for a drug.

---

### DOSAGE

The dosage available varies country by country. In the UK, the standard dosage is 300mg and 75mg for the low dose variety.

In the USA, it is available as 325mg and 85mg for the low dose form. It is said that the American version relates to the old system of dosage, in which drugs were supplied in grains. Five grains of ASA were equivalent to 325mg. It is also suggested that this size of tablet gave just enough room to have 'Bayer' stamped on it.

The difference in these doses is not medically significant.

In that same year, Bayer started distributing it to doctors in powder form, urging them to try it on their patients.

In 1915, Aspirin became available in tablet form for the first time. It also became obtainable over the counter without a doctor's prescription. It rapidly became the most commonly used drug in the world. By 1920, it was promoted and used as an effective drug for rheumatism, lumbago and neuralgia.

## Aspirin in wartime

During the First World War, there was concern among the Allies that they would run out of aspirin, as they obviously would not have access to supplies from Germany.

Accordingly, the British government offered a reward of £20,000 to anyone who could come up with an alternative method of manufacture. The Australian pharmacist George Nicholas developed a method and patented his version as Aspro in Melbourne in 1915.

The 1918 flu pandemic, which came at the end of the First World War and which resulted in the deaths of between 20 and 40 million people worldwide, was the trigger for widespread use of aspirin. While aspirin was not a cure for the deadly strain of flu, and could not prevent the deaths the flu caused, the drug nevertheless became established as a popular treatment for colds and feverish illnesses, and proved itself effective at treating the symptoms of such conditions.

## A brilliant deduction

Following the Second World War, in 1948, Dr Lawrence Craven, a Californian GP and Ear, Nose and Throat specialist, started giving a type of chewing gum impregnated with aspirin, called Aspergum, to his patients after tonsillectomies.

He noted that those people who used an excessive amount developed complications with bleeding. He conjectured that aspirin was interfering with their ability to clot their blood.

From this conjecture, it was a short step for Craven to theorize whether the drug could prevent people developing blood clots in their coronary arteries: a cause of a heart attack. He started to prescribe aspirin in low doses – and found that over a follow-up period of several years, he recorded a significantly lower rate of both heart attacks and strokes.

Craven published several papers in obscure medical journals rather than the prominent ones, and his findings were not taken up by the medical profession. It is not known whether he had attempted to submit his work to the main journals first.

### ASPIRIN AND CHILDREN

In 1952, children's chewable aspirin was introduced. This was a low dose preparation, which was used continuously until 1979, when research by Dr Karen Starko in Phoenix, Arizona, found a significant link between aspirin and Reye's syndrome, a potentially fatal condition in children. Since then, aspirin is not prescribed to anyone under the age of sixteen years.

## Aspirin's amazing secrets revealed

The latter part of the last century saw huge advances in our understanding of the potential of aspirin, thanks to the efforts of a wide range of research studies. It became clear that the drug had a much broader and more significant reach than anyone had ever anticipated. While the drug may have been named for the patron saint of headaches, aspirin's impact was quickly shown to be effective in far more serious complaints – triumphing against even fatal conditions.

- In 1974, Professor Peter Elwood of the MRC (Medical Research Council) Epidemiology Unit in South Wales performed the first trial of aspirin in the prevention of heart attacks. Patients who had already had a heart attack were randomly allocated to receive one type of treatment or another; in this case, either active aspirin or placebo (a 'fake' drug which has no effect). The trial showed that aspirin reduced mortality by 24 per cent.
- In the 1970s, pharmacologist Professor John Vane discovered exactly how aspirin worked, namely by blocking an enzyme involved in prostaglandin production. The prostaglandins are important natural hormones that are involved in many body processes, including pain, tissue injury and inflammation. The way in which aspirin interacts with them is crucial in explaining how aspirin works, which we'll look at in detail in chapter 4.
- In 1989, a preliminary pilot study in the USA suggested that aspirin could delay the onset of dementia.
- In 1995, researchers in the USA suggested that aspirin had some protective function against cancer of the bowel.
- In 1998, the Medical Research Council's Thrombosis Prevention Trial demonstrated that both low dose aspirin and low dose warfarin (a drug that prevents blood clotting, called an 'anticoagulant') reduced the incidence of a heart attack in men at high risk, and that when the two agents were combined, the reduction in risk was even greater.

## Aspirin in the twenty-first century

The dawn of a new millennium didn't stop aspirin's seemingly unstoppable rise to acclaim. In fact, the results now coming in – and they will continue to do so, as many studies are taking place across the world even as I write – are even more extraordinary than all the facts known up to this point.

One example concerns the second biggest killer of humankind: cancer. Amazingly, in 2010, a major review from Oxford University and other centres, covering over 25,000 patients, found that a small daily dose of aspirin could reduce the overall cancer death rate by at least one fifth.

## The research goes on

In July 2010, the University of Pittsburgh in the USA began recruiting patients for a new prospective study to see whether aspirin can actually prolong life and prevent physical debility and dementia in healthy older people.

The Aspirin in Reducing Events in the Elderly (ASPREE) study will be a large international trial covering 6,500 patients of 70 years and over in the USA and 12,500 of the same age in Australia.[2] It will run for at least 5 years, when we can expect to hear about its results.

# HOW ASPIRIN WORKS

## 4

As you might expect, the mechanisms by which aspirin works are fairly complex to explain. Consequently, I have deliberately tried to avoid difficult scientific descriptions and too much extraneous background information in this chapter.

This chapter aims to explain in reasonably simple terms the mechanisms that make aspirin such an effective drug.

## Chemical make-up

As drugs go, aspirin is a very simple chemical molecule. You would not expect this to be the case in a drug that has been shown to have such a wide range of effects.

The formula of aspirin is $C_9H_8O_4$.

The structure of aspirin is:

Note the part of the structure in bold. This denotes the acetyl group, which – as you may remember – was added to the base form of aspirin (salicylic acid) by aspirin's creators. This structure is highly important. Neither of aspirin's creators – neither Charles Frederic Gerhardt in 1853, nor Felix Hoffman in 1897 – realized that by 'buffering' salicylic acid by adding the acetyl (which they did to protect the stomach) they had enormously boosted the drug's potential.

# The pioneers

The scientists primarily responsible for our present understanding of aspirin are Professor John Vane and Priscilla Piper. They were to make a discovery that would earn John Vane both a Nobel Prize in medicine and physiology, and a knighthood.

The breakthrough Vane and Piper made was in finding that if tissue was treated with aspirin, then it inhibited the release of what are called 'prostaglandins'.

### What's a prostaglandin?

Prostaglandins are compounds made in the body from fatty acids. The Swedish physiologist Ulf von Euler first isolated them from secretions of the prostate gland in 1935, hence the name they were given.

They are in fact produced in most tissues and organs of the body. They are messenger compounds that have a great variety of functions.

- Some of the functions are helpful and protective to the body, such as regulating the kidney function, protecting the stomach and controlling cell growth.
- Some effects are decidedly unwanted, such as causing bronchospasm (spasm of the airways in the lungs, like in

asthma), anaphylactic reactions, excessive inflammation and pain.

## What effect do prostaglandins have?

A variety of effects can happen when prostaglandins are released. Exactly which effects will result depends upon which prostaglandins are released and which part of the body they are released in.

Prostaglandins can:

- Regulate kidney function
- Control cell growth
- Sensitize nerve cells to pain
- Raise body temperature during infections
- Protect the stomach from its own acid
- Regulate menstrual function in females
- Help to heal injuries by promoting inflammation
- Dilate or constrict blood vessels
- Cause smooth muscle to relax or contract
- Affect the pressure within the eye

And much more.

# The first key discovery

Vane and Piper discovered that the prostaglandins causing pain and inflammation were blocked by aspirin; hence the drug's effectiveness in treating these conditions.

The same results were also observed with two other drugs, sodium salicylate and indomethacin, both of which are Non-Steroidal Anti-Inflammatory Drugs (NSAIDs), the family of drugs to which aspirin belongs. There was no such effect with other drugs such as morphine.

Vane published his results in *Nature* in 1971.[3]

## Supportive evidence

In the same issue of *Nature*, another paper was published by another team working in the same department.[4] This was independent of Vane's study, and was a study of the effects of aspirin on the behaviour of platelets (the smallest blood cells).

Unlike Vane's experiments, which were conducted on animal tissue, this was done on humans. Volunteers were given aspirin, then blood samples were checked to look at their platelets to measure the blood levels of various substances, including prostaglandins. The researchers found that when aspirin had been given, the levels of prostaglandins were reduced.

This helped to confirm John Vane's theory.

## The full picture

John Vane's breakthrough discovery was followed by several other discoveries which all helped to build up the full picture of how aspirin worked, like the pieces of a jigsaw.

To understand this, we first need to look at what happens if tissue is damaged. It's best to imagine this as a kind of chain reaction in the body, kickstarted by damaged cells.

### Step one

When a cell is damaged – for example, by injury or infection – it releases a substance known as arachidonic acid. Nothing to do with spiders: it's an essential fatty acid that is an integral component of cell membranes.

### Step two

An enzyme called cyclo-oxygenase (known as COX, like the apple) then converts the arachidonic acid into these prostaglandins we've already read so much about.

Three types of COX have been discovered. They are each responsible for converting the different kinds of prostaglandins: so some look after the 'nice' prostaglandins (those that protect the stomach) while others have a hand in the 'nasty' ones (those that cause inflammation). The three types of COX are as follows:

- **COX-1** – is present throughout the whole body all the time at low levels. It is involved in keeping up a small supply of prostaglandins to maintain bodily functions. It has a protective function with the stomach and intestines.
- **COX-2** – becomes active as a response to infection or damage to cells. It tends to promote inflammatory changes, the rise in body temperature of fever, and be involved in the sensation of pain.
- **COX-3** – its function has not been fully elucidated as yet. It is present in the brain and may have a role in headaches.

## Aspirin in action

Scientists have found that aspirin inhibits the action of both the COX-2 and COX-1 enzymes. This accounts for both its benefits and its side effects.

- Most of the beneficial effects of aspirin appear to derive from its inactivation of the COX-2 enzyme.
- The side effects of aspirin seem to arise because it inactivates the beneficial role of the COX-1 enzyme.

The acetyl group of the aspirin molecule (the bold section of the chemical diagram on page 45) is responsible for part of this inhibitive effect. It binds to a receptor site (it *acetylates*, to use the technical term) on the COX-1 or COX-2 enzyme and blocks its action permanently.

To put this in simpler terms, you may think of the receptor

site of the COX enzyme as being like a lock, and the arachidonic acid being like a key. What happens when we take aspirin is that the acetyl group in aspirin blocks the lock, so the arachidonic acid can't slot into the site – which means the reaction doesn't take place. Aspirin 'locks' the enzyme up. The COX enzymes cannot then engage with the arachidonic acid, so the rest of the reaction to produce prostaglandins cannot take place.

## The benefits

Many of aspirin's benefits arise from its ability to block COX-2. The COX-2 enzyme is the one that comes into action during tissue injury, illness and infection. So in blocking its effects, aspirin:

- Reduces pain by stopping prostaglandins from increasing the sensitivity of nerve cells.
- Reduces inflammation by stopping prostaglandins producing and boosting other mediators of inflammation.
- Reduces fever by blocking a prostaglandin that directly stimulates the body's temperature-control centre in the brain (this stimulation causes the body temperature to rise during infections, so the lack of stimulation means body temperature remains normal).
- Allows the blood vessels to dilate to dissipate body heat.

## Side effects

The COX-1 enzyme, on the other hand, causes the body to keep up its level of *beneficial* prostaglandins. So in blocking COX-1, aspirin can have a negative effect for some patients. For example:

- The most common complaint from patients who have problems with aspirin is to do with stomach irritation. This involves the hydrochloric acid your stomach produces to help you digest your food. It is an extremely powerful acid, but the lining of the stomach is normally protected by a layer of bicarbonate and mucus. This layer is stimulated by prostaglandins that are created by the action of COX-1. So if the enzyme is inhibited, this protective layer is not maintained – and all manner of complications can ensue, from simple inflammation to ulceration or even bleeding.
- The smooth muscle control is affected, so that bronchospasm may occur – causing asthma attacks and breathing difficulties.
- The kidney tissue may be affected to reduce its function and flow of urine, resulting in kidney troubles.

---

### ASPIRIN IN GOUT

Aspirin's effect on the kidneys may explain its beneficial effect in treating gout. The problem in gout is defective metabolism of uric acid, often resulting in the body having too much uric acid.

Aspirin reduces the kidney's ability to reabsorb uric acid from the blood that passes through its special system of tubules. In so doing, it enables the kidneys to get rid of excess uric acid by putting it into the urine, which is eventually passed by the patient. Thus the uric acid levels in the body decrease, thereby helping the gout.

## The problem of bleeding

The tendency to bleed comes about because aspirin also affects the COX-1 enzyme that is carried on each little platelet in the blood.

The platelets are the smallest of all the blood cells, their function being to clump together to produce a blood clot to seal off tiny blood vessels when there has been injury to a tissue. The COX-1 enzyme in the platelet is responsible for transforming a prostaglandin called Prostaglandin H into a substance called thromboxane-2. Thromboxane causes the platelets to be sticky, which enables them to clot together more easily.

When COX-1 is inhibited by aspirin and reduces the production of thomboxane, platelet stickiness is reduced (so wounds cannot heal as easily) and there is a tendency to increased bruising and bleeding.

While this reduced platelet stickiness can be a dreadful side effect for some, it actually helps patients at risk of cardiovascular disease by reducing the chance of a blood clot forming in the coronary or cerebral arteries, and therefore reducing the risk of a heart attack or stroke.

---

### THE LIFE OF A PLATELET

A platelet lives for only about 7 or 8 days. Aspirin will cause a platelet to lose its ability to clot for the duration of its life. A platelet is a unique type of cell which does not have a nucleus containing DNA, therefore it is unable to manufacture more COX-1. This means that after you take an aspirin tablet, your platelets will be less sticky than they were before you took the aspirin, and the effect will persist for a week.

## A drug without side effects?

As you would expect, there is ongoing research to see whether someone can safely develop a drug that only inhibits COX-2 and leaves the beneficial COX-1 alone.

There have been some selective COX-2 inhibitors which seemed to be very effective in reducing inflammation, pain and fevers without producing stomach problems. Unfortunately, after eighteen months of usage, they seemed to be associated with an increased incidence of cardiovascular events – strokes, heart attacks and thrombosis. Research continues in order to find a selective COX-2 inhibitor that can be taken long term.

## Other effects

Research has shown that, as well as blocking the COX enzymes, aspirin also has other effects in the body, such as:

- Stimulating natural chemicals called resolvins, which shut down the body's inflammatory response (these are discussed in the next chapter).
- Forming nitric oxide radicals or NO-radicals, which may be important in the condition of depression (examined in Chapter 16).

## Low dose aspirin

We shall see in the following chapters that aspirin in low dose, a 75mg tablet a day, seems to have remarkable powers in reducing the risk of developing some major diseases.

Although we have an appreciation of how aspirin blocks the different COX enzymes, it is not entirely clear how it produces its beneficial effects in the long term. It may be that, in terms of reducing the risk of cardiovascular disease, its ability to block COX-1 to reduce platelet stickiness is the main mechanism. On the other hand, its ability to reduce the risk of cancer may be mainly to do with its ability to block COX-2. Some research suggests that both are important at the same time.

In preventing major diseases, aspirin seems to be working by a different mechanism than it does when taken at standard dosage to reduce pain, inflammation and fevers. Larger doses are needed for these more immediate effects, whereas the long-term effects that only require low doses seem to be altogether subtler.

Clearly, aspirin has not yet revealed all of its secrets. Another Nobel prize may await whoever fathoms them out.

# PAIN, FEVER AND INFLAMMATION

As we discussed in chapter 3 on the History of Aspirin, its use from the days of the ancient Sumerians illustrates the convoluted way in which medicine advances.

In its crude form of willow bark, it was empirically discovered by various cultures around the world and found to be effective in the treatment of the three fundamental areas that matter to people during illness:

- Pain
- Fever
- Inflammation

These are still as important to us today as they were then.

## PAIN

This is the single most common symptom that alerts people to the fact that they have a problem or that they need to take action to remove themselves from a source of danger.

There are many types of pain and many different causes.

- A broken bone will cause excruciating pain and will require a significant pain reliever.

- A sore throat will produce a very uncomfortable pain, which may be dealt with by warm drinks and gargles.
- Appendicitis will produce extreme abdominal pain, which must not be suppressed with painkillers, but necessitates a surgical operation to remove the inflamed organ.
- A heart attack causes agonizing central chest pain which can radiate to other parts of the body, e.g. down one's arm.

Already, one can see that pain is no simple matter. Very different pathological processes can cause the unpleasant experience that we call pain. There is no doubt that pain is an enigma.

Happily, nowadays we have a much better understanding about the enigma of pain, which is helping us to develop different strategies to manage the different types.

## Types of pain

It is important to differentiate acute from chronic pain. These are not words used to express two poles of a spectrum of experience. They are two entirely different types of pain.

- **Acute pain** is the expected physiological response to a stimulation, which is immediately perceived as being potentially damaging and highly unpleasant to the body. The simplest example is the immediate reflex withdrawal of your hand when you burn your fingers. If the burn is mild, the pain will go in a relatively short period of time. This type of pain is seen to have a purpose, in that it alerts the body to a problem that it can readily relieve. It causes the individual to take action to avoid further injury or damage.

- **Chronic pain** is the continual experience of an unpleasant sensation, which is unlikely to disappear of its own accord. This is the typical background chronic pain of arthritis or the type that can occur with some types of neuralgia (inflamed nerve pain). It also occurs when there is pressure on a nerve to cause nerve root irritation, as in sciatica. This pain has no useful function.

- **Recurrent pain** is the term used to describe acute pain that occurs in repeated episodes. This is the type that you get with repeated episodes of irritable bowel syndrome or bouts of back pain.

Acute pain is usually treatable with painkillers and anti-inflammatory agents. Chronic pain can be far harder to control just with these drugs, and other strategies need to be adopted.

## How aspirin works ... as a painkiller

The work of Professor Sir John Vane showed us that aspirin works by blocking the action of the COX enzyme system. This reduces production of prostaglandins, many of which are mediators of inflammation, and which stimulate the sensors that send the pain signal along nerves. Put very simply:

no prostaglandins = no signal sent that you're feeling pain = no pain

Though it is not quite as simple as that, of course. Prostaglandins are among the main mediators of inflammation – but there are others. Aspirin will not affect them, so they may continue to produce some pain signal. However, the net effect of aspirin will have been to reduce the pain level.

The dosage needed to achieve pain relief of headaches, menstrual pain, rheumatic or arthritic pain is usually 300–900mg every 4 to 6 hours, as is found to be necessary. The maximum dosage in any 24 hours is 4g.

It is necessary to take these high doses in order to achieve a therapeutic blood level. That means a sufficient amount of the drug in the blood in order to exert an effect on the tissues that are causing the pain.

It will also reduce pain through its anti-inflammatory effect, since this will reduce the production of prostaglandins that cause swelling of the tissues and irritation around blood vessels. We shall consider this in the next section on inflammation. It is just as important to appreciate that this is part of the painkilling effect.

It also seems that aspirin has a central or direct effect on the brain and the central nervous system. It is possible that it could have an effect on COX-3 in the brain, but further research will be needed to elucidate or refute this.

## FEVER

The word fever comes from the Latin *fervere*, meaning 'to be hot, to boil'. Feverish illnesses have always been common and there are many causes.

A rise in body temperature is one of the manifestations of inflammation somewhere in the body. If the temperature rises too high, then it can cause cerebral or brain irritation, which can result in a convulsion.

## Treating a fever

Early doctors had observed these convulsions, yet were not aware of their significance. Their medical texts taught that fevers should be burned out of the system by the use of steam, warm blankets and getting the temperature of the sick room up. The idea was to try to bring an illness to a crisis, that is, to a peak in temperature, after which the body would recover.

Later, more enlightened doctors taught that one should do whatever one could to bring the temperature down, using cooling swabs and baths, and also medicines that had the

PAIN, FEVER AND INFLAMMATION

ability to reduce the temperature. Such remedies were called febrifuges, from the Latin *febris*, meaning 'burning', and *fugere*, meaning 'to flee or drive away'.

## Aspirin to the rescue

Willow was considered a powerful febrifuge.

Later, once we had a better understanding of the causes and the effects of a fever in illness, and of the importance of body temperature, the word pyrexia was used in medicine instead of fever, and the drugs that could lower the pyrexia (from the Greek *pyrexis*, meaning 'feverishness') were termed anti-pyretics.

Here again, one of the most effective anti-pyretic drugs was none other than aspirin.

## How aspirin works ... to reduce temperature

The fact that aspirin was found to be good at reducing abnormal high temperatures, such as occur in infectious diseases, yet had no effect on normal temperatures always seemed paradoxical.

A part of the brain called the hypothalamus is responsible for controlling heart rate and body temperature. When the body temperature gets too high, the hypothalamus takes action to cause perspiration and dilation of blood vessels in the skin to effect loss of heat. However, in many illnesses, prostaglandins reduce the hypothalamus's ability to do this, and so the temperature rises.

We now know of course that aspirin reduces the production of prostaglandins, thereby allowing the hypothalamus to lower the temperature as it is intended to do. This is why it will not reduce it below normal.

# INFLAMMATION

As we saw in chapter 3 on the History of Aspirin, Aulus Cornelius Celsus, a Roman encyclopaedist writing in the first century AD, described the four cardinal signs of inflammation in his book *De Medicina*. The signs of *calor* (warmth), *dolor* (pain), *tumor* (swelling) and *rubor* (heat) are still regarded as cardinal clinical signs of inflammation. This means that they are the outward signs that a doctor can pick up on in a physical examination.

Inflammation seems to be part of the cause of many chronic conditions, as we shall see in subsequent chapters.

## What is inflammation?

The inflammatory response is a natural mechanism whereby the body tries to repair damage or to remove infection. In the case of a simple spot, for example, invading microorganisms have entered the skin and they attempt to overcome the body's defences by reproducing themselves rapidly. The body mobilizes its defences, involving blood cells, which accumulate in large volumes and produce a creamy fluid that is called pus.

Thus the spot gradually rises, the area goes red and it feels hot and painful. When it 'comes to a head', it means that there is a collection of pus under the skin. This will either discharge outwards or the body will continue to fight the infection until it overcomes it. This causes the inflammation to spread into the surrounding tissue. Once the body overcomes the infection, the inflammatory response will close down, resulting in the swelling lessening, the redness and heat going, and the pain disappearing.

The body's inflammatory response can be simply summarized as follows:

# PAIN, FEVER AND INFLAMMATION

- Injury or infection causes increased blood flow to the affected area – which can sometimes produce a visible redness on the skin, and increased heat to the touch.
- Fluid rich in white blood cells and special natural chemicals will ooze from the blood vessels into the tissues to surround the damaged cells at the entrance to infection. This results in swelling of the affected area and in the case of infection, the accumulation of pus.
- Stimulation of pain sensors in the area by prostaglandins and other substances.
- The inflammatory response will continue until it is signalled to close down.

The problem with the inflammatory response is that once it is started, it can be hard to control. You can liken it to using a military tank rather than a postal van to deliver mail. It overdoes the job and it may cause more damage and more distress than is necessary.

This is where medicine comes in. Its purpose is to reduce excess damage and distress. From your reading of chapter 4, you can see how aspirin will help. In particular, it can assist by blocking prostaglandin production. Prostaglandin types 2, especially PG E2, are powerful mediators of inflammation.

## Closing inflammation down

The inflammatory response will continue until all invading organisms have been removed and the tissue is repaired or healed as well as it can be. Sometimes, of course, it will go on for longer than necessary if the body has somehow developed antibodies to itself and a chronic inflammatory process has begun.

This unstoppable inflammation may be part of the cause of many chronic conditions, as we shall discuss in later chapters. Generally, however, the body will close down the inflammatory response when it is not needed.

This closing down of the response is called inflammatory resolution.

## How aspirin works ... as an anti-inflammatory

We have already seen that aspirin works by blocking production of prostaglandins, so it will have a general effect on reducing inflammation. In addition to this general effect, it also seems to help directly in closing down the inflammatory response.

A group of chemicals called, appropriately enough, resolvins act to resolve the body's inflammatory response. Aspirin seems to stimulate the production of resolvins, thereby helping to close down the inflammatory response – thus reducing swelling, heat and pain.

## Anti-inflammatory drugs

Our increasing knowledge about what goes on at the cellular level has allowed us to develop ever more powerful anti-inflammatory drugs.

Aspirin was the very first of the Non-Steroidal Anti-Inflammatory Drugs (NSAIDs) to be discovered.

While there are other drugs with greater anti-inflammatory ability than aspirin, its broad-ranging effects on the COX enzyme system and on the resolvins is of inestimable importance in producing many of its many beneficial effects on health – and its ability to prevent many serious medical conditions.

## ASPIRIN IN PRACTICE

So far we have been talking about pain, fever and inflammation in a general sense. It is now worth looking at some scientific studies that have been done to demonstrate how people feel when they are treated for real conditions with aspirin.

## Aspirin for sore throats and colds

The common cold is generally regarded as a trivial complaint, although it causes a great deal of misery, and loss of time from work. In addition, it diminishes people's resistance and it creates the right conditions for patients to get more serious secondary infections of the sinuses and the chest.

It is a good example of a condition that causes pain, fever and inflammation. It should, therefore, be eminently suitable for the administration of aspirin.

In 2003, the Common Cold Centre at the University of Cardiff conducted a placebo-controlled, double-blind-controlled study on aspirin's effect on sore throat and other painful symptoms during colds in the UK and in Sweden.[5] 'Double-blind-controlled' means that patients were at random given one of two types of treatment and that neither the patients *nor* the researchers knew which they were given. In this case, patients were given either an active treatment or a placebo treatment.

- 272 patients with cold symptoms were recruited onto the trial. The average age was 25 years and 109 were male, 163 were female.
- They were asked to grade their throat pain on a scale of 0–10.
- 60–70 per cent had additional symptoms of headache, sneezing and a runny nose.
- 53 per cent had nasal congestion.
- 45 per cent had muscle pains.
- They were randomly chosen to receive either a single dose of 800mg aspirin and 480mg Vitamin C or a placebo.

- Symptoms were monitored for 2 hours in clinic and for 4 hours by the patients at home.

### The results

- The researchers found that aspirin significantly reduced pain intensity and there was a 20–30 per cent difference between the two groups.
- The main effect was apparent at 2 hours and lasted for 5 hours.
- There were no significant adverse effects that could be separated from the symptoms associated with a cold, and there was no difference found between the two groups.

### Conclusion

Aspirin is an effective treatment for the sore throat, headache and muscle pain associated with the common cold.

## Aspirin and headaches

Headaches are very common and the majority are not serious. The two most common types of headache are tension headaches and migraine.

### Tension headaches

These are extremely common. In any year, 86 per cent of women and 63 per cent of men will experience a tension headache.[6]

As the name implies, these headaches are due to muscle tension in the scalp. This is usually due to stress and tends to be amenable to painkillers.

One placebo-controlled study on the use of aspirin for tension headache found that the dose has to be adequate for the drug to have an effect.[7] This means that the higher the dose, the greater number of people experienced relief. The response rates:

- 75.7 per cent at 1,000mg aspirin experienced relief.
- 70.3 per cent at 500mg aspirin experienced relief.
- 54.5 per cent with placebo experienced relief.

## Migraine

A lot of people think that migraine is simply a strong headache. It is in fact a vascular headache, caused by dilation of the blood vessels within the scalp and the skull. Many migraine sufferers experience an aura before the headache comes on. This tends to be due to vaso-constriction or spasm of the blood vessels before they dilate. It produces visual disturbance, light-headedness and nausea. Then when the blood vessels dilate, the pain comes.

About 20 per cent of women experience migraines and 10 per cent of men.

## Can aspirin help with migraine?

In 2005, the effectiveness of aspirin in a single attack of migraine was investigated in a placebo-controlled, double-blind parallel study.[8] A single dose of aspirin or placebo was given at the start of a migraine.

There was a significant difference found between the two groups and the authors concluded that aspirin was an effective and safe treatment for migraine in appropriately selected patients.

Today, BASH, the British Association for the Study of Headache, recommends that migraine sufferers take over-the-counter (OTC) painkillers in the first instance.

**CHAPTER SUMMARY**

Aspirin is one of the most effective drugs in our medical arsenal for reducing pain, fever and inflammation. Used in full dose as an active treatment for evident medical problems, it has been proven to help with such conditions as headaches, the common cold, menstrual pain, arthritis and rheumatism. If you're feeling ill with such symptoms, aspirin is an excellent over-the-counter drug to take, provided of course that your medical history allows you to use it.

# 6
# THE HEART AND CIRCULATION

The circulatory system consists of the heart and the blood vessels that carry blood around the body to all of its organs and tissues. In this chapter, we'll be looking at how this system works, what can go wrong (the causes of heart attacks), and how aspirin has been shown to prevent not only second heart attacks, but also primary attacks.

## Statistics – the heart of the matter

- In 2011, there are estimated to be 1.1 million men with angina in the UK. (Angina is explained on page 76.)
- 6.5 per cent of men have heart disease in the UK.
- 4 per cent of women have heart disease in the UK.
- The rate rises with age. One in three men and one in four women over the age of 75 years will have heart disease.
- Men are 2–3 times more at risk than women *until* the menopause. The female hormones seem to have a protective effect and after the menopause that protective role is lost, so the rates are then far closer.
- Heart and circulatory diseases are the UK's biggest killer. In 2007, cardiovascular disease caused 34 per cent of the deaths in the UK (193,000 people).

- According to the Scottish Continuous Morbidity Study, there are a total of 96,000 new cases of angina per year.
- The cost of healthcare in the UK as the result of cardiovascular disease is £1.7 billion per year.

> **Cardiovascular disease** means disease affecting the heart and the blood vessels. It can result in heart attacks, strokes and death.
>
> **Coronary artery disease** specifically refers to problems with the supply of blood to the heart, primarily through blocked arteries.

### How can aspirin help?

Before we can answer that question, we need to look at what a heart attack is, and the key causes of cardiovascular disease. But first, we need to understand the heart and the circulatory system itself: the very thing that keeps us all alive.

## The heart

- The heart is a hollow muscular pump.
- It has four chambers: two upper ones called the atria, which pass blood into the two lower chambers, called the ventricles.
- Effectively, the heart is like two pumps joined together; the left side of the heart receives oxygenated (oxygen-rich) blood from the lungs and pumps it out to the tissues. This is called *the systemic circulation*.
- The right side receives deoxygenated (oxygen-depleted)

## THE HEART AND CIRCULATION

blood from the tissues and pumps it out to the lungs to collect more oxygen. This is called *the pulmonary circulation*.

- There are four valves in the heart, whose purpose is to ensure that blood flows through the heart in the right direction between the four chambers.

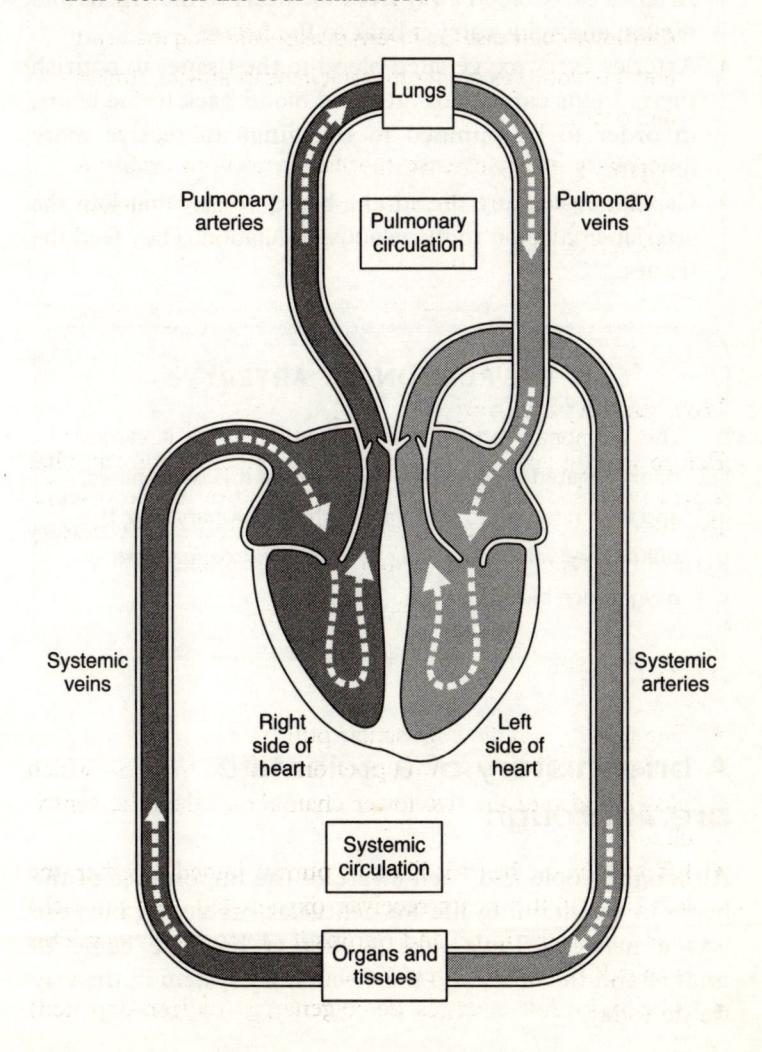

## The blood vessels

There are three types of blood vessel: arteries, veins and capillaries.

- Arteries carry blood away from the heart to the organs and tissues, and veins carry it back to the heart.
- Arteries carry oxygenated blood to the tissues to nourish them. Veins carry deoxygenated blood back to the heart, in order to be pumped to the lungs to receive more oxygen.
- Capillaries are tiny thread-like blood vessels that join the arterial circulation to the venous circulation. They feed the tissues.

> **THE PULMONARY ARTERY**
>
> The pulmonary artery is an exception, since it carries deoxygenated blood to the lungs where it is oxygenated, and then returned to the heart by the pulmonary vein. The pulmonary vein is the only vein to carry oxygenated or oxygen-rich blood.

## A brief history of a scientific breakthrough

Although people had been aware of the importance of the heart in maintaining life for centuries, its actual purpose was a mystery. Let's take a look at how we came to understand the heart and the circulatory system in the way we do today.

## The first theory

Anatomists like Andreas Vesalius (1514–64) had observed that there was a difference between the blood in arteries and the blood in veins. He thought that the heart manufactured arterial blood and that the liver manufactured venous blood, both types being sent to the extremities of the body by some sort of sucking mechanism of the heart and the liver. When the blood reached its target, it was used up.

## The work of William Harvey

William Harvey (1578–1657) was a physician and anatomist who fought in the English Civil War and who was court physician to three kings of England. After graduating from Cambridge University, he went to study medicine and anatomy at the University of Padua.

He did not think that the idea of blood being manufactured by the heart and the liver was logical. Simple arithmetic showed that a huge amount of blood would have to be produced and used up in a short period of time.

After extensive experimentation on animals, Harvey came to the conclusion that there was a constant amount of blood, and that it was in continual circulation, pumped by the heart through the blood vessels.

## The breakthrough

Harvey announced his discovery of the circulation of the blood in 1616, and in 1628 he published his work *Exercitatio Anatomica de Motu Cordis et Sanguinis in Animalibus* (An Anatomical Exercise on the Motion of the Heart and Blood in Animals). It was the most significant piece of medical research ever written and laid the foundation for the scientific study of medicine.

He proposed that blood flowed through the heart in two separate loops, a pulmonary circulation going to the lungs and another, the system circulation, going to the organs and extremities.

### Fabricius

Harvey's work in Padua under another anatomist known as Fabricius helped him to understand the function of the valves in veins. They only work in one direction, so Harvey concluded that they were designed to allow blood to flow towards the heart, but *not* in the other direction. This suggested that the blood flowed around and around the body and that the two circulations were in some way linked.

### Marcello Malpighi

In 1661, Marcello Malpighi (1628–94), an Italian doctor, published the results of his experiments on the microscopic examination of the anatomy of a frog's lung. He reported on his findings of *capillaries*, the tiny blood vessels that link the arteries to the veins. This was the missing link that Harvey had been looking for. The complete circulation of the blood had been discovered.

## The lining of the blood vessels

Almost without exception, the blood vessels are lined with a single layer of flat cells called epithelial cells. The lining is referred to as the epithelium. It is smooth in good health.

This lining can become damaged if the state of arteriosclerosis develops. This is also known as hardening of the arteries, and is a major cause of heart disease.

## The blood

There are about ten pints of blood in the average adult. It makes up roughly one eleventh or about 9 per cent of the body weight. It is composed of:

- A fluid called plasma, which is 91 per cent water and 9 per cent solids and other contents – proteins, salts, digested products, waste products, carried oxygen and carbon dioxide gases, hormones, enzymes and various messenger chemicals.
- Blood cells:
  o Red blood cells, which carry the oxygen.
  o White blood cells, of various types, which fight infection and protect the body.
  o Platelets, which clump together to produce clots to plug any breaches in blood vessels.

## The blood supply to the heart

This is the part that surprises many people. The heart has ten pints of blood flowing through it all the time, yet the condition of *angina* comes about when the heart is temporarily deprived of oxygen. Worse, if part of the heart is deprived completely of oxygen-rich blood for long, then a heart attack may be the result.

The question is: why can't the heart get its oxygen directly from the blood that flows through it?

The reason is that the heart is made up of muscle tissue called the *myocardium*. It has to be given its oxygen – and all the other nutrients that the blood supplies – in exactly the same way as every other tissue of the body: it has to receive it from the capillaries that run through it. And they in turn have to be supplied by their own arteries.

**AN ASPIRIN A DAY**

## The coronary arteries

The coronary arteries are the blood vessels that directly supply the heart. If problems arise in any of these arteries, in short, you're in trouble. Yet as we will find out later in this chapter (see page 81), which artery is affected has a crucial impact on a patient's prognosis – and even influences whether you are more likely to live or die.

There are two main coronary arteries, the left coronary artery and the right coronary artery. They both arise from the main blood vessel, the aorta, soon after it leaves the heart from the left ventricle. Each coronary artery supplies a different part of the heart with oxygenated blood.

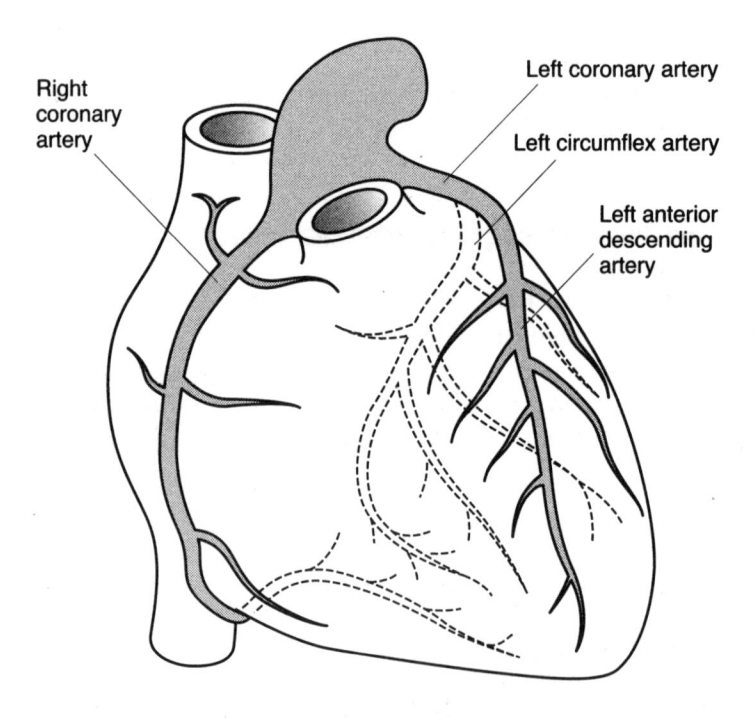

- Right coronary artery – supplies oxygenated blood to the walls of the ventricles and the right atrium.

- Left coronary artery – carries oxygenated blood and divides into two vessels:
  - Left anterior descending artery – supplies the walls of the ventricles and the left atrium. Essentially, it supplies the front of the heart.
  - Left circumflex artery – supplies blood to the walls of the ventricles and the left atrium. Essentially, it supplies the back of the heart.

## What can go wrong with the heart?

There are four basic things that can go wrong with the heart:

1. It can beat in an abnormal rhythm (e.g. atrial fibrillation, see page 76).
2. It can be temporarily deprived of oxygen to produce an anginal attack.
3. It can be totally deprived of oxygen for so long (and it only takes a few minutes) to produce death of part of the heart muscle. This is called a *myocardial infarction*. A myocardial infarction is the most common form of what we generally call a 'heart attack', and for reasons of simplicity I will refer to this condition as a 'heart attack' from here on in.
4. The heart can stop. This is called a cardiac arrest. If the heart does not restart spontaneously, or is not made to restart by CPR or with an electrical shock, then death results.

Coronary artery disease is often (but not always) the cause of all of these.

Now let's look at each of the potential problems in more detail.

### Abnormal rhythms

The heart beats regularly throughout health. Each beat is initiated by the heart's natural pacemaker, the sino-atrial node, which is situated in the right atrium.

Certain conditions result in the natural pacemaker not working correctly, so that other parts of the heart may take up the pacemaker role. These other pacemakers may do so erratically, causing irregularity of the heartbeat. Sometimes this will cause it to race and produce the sensation of palpitations, and sometimes it may cause it to go slow, so that it does not work efficiently.

The main causes are:

- Certain heart valve problems
- Overactive thyroid gland
- Coronary artery disease resulting in blocked arteries and a lack of blood flow to the heart

---

### ATRIAL FIBRILLATION

*Atrial fibrillation* is a condition in which the atria contract repeatedly, totally out of phase with the ventricles, so that the heart beats very irregularly. As a result, the pumping may not be efficient enough to oxygenate the blood and the individual may feel tired and breathless.

Of even more significance, the irregular beating predisposes to clot formation within the heart. If such a clot is produced, it may work its way via the circulation system to the brain and cause one type of stroke called an *ischaemic stroke*. We shall look at this further in the next chapter.

---

### Angina pectoris

This is the name for a pain in the chest that arises from narrowing of the coronary arteries, usually from coronary artery disease.

## THE HEART AND CIRCULATION

- It classically produces central chest pain with radiation of pain down the left arm to the hand.
- It is usually precipitated by exercise and is relieved by rest.
- A history of angina dramatically increases the risk of a heart attack.
- Angina pectoris should always be thoroughly investigated and should be treated with appropriate medication.

> ### ACUTE CORONARY SYNDROME
>
> Unstable angina, that is angina that is occurring often and unpredictably, and heart attacks are both included in acute coronary syndrome (ACS). They are all the result of *myocardial ischaemia*, meaning lack of oxygen to the heart muscle.

## Myocardial infarction (MI)

This is generally what is described as a heart attack. MI is the name given to death of part of the heart muscle as the result of a diminished blood supply and oxygen deprivation to it.

A heart attack is always serious:

- About 240,000 people have a heart attack in England and Wales every year.
- 50 per cent of those who die from a heart attack do so within the first hour.
- Death is commonly due to an abnormal rhythm being provoked.
- The risk of death declines hour by hour.
- Emergency treatment is essential, including the immediate use of aspirin and access to a defibrillator if necessary.

There are several complications of such heart attacks, all of which need to be investigated and treated vigorously:

- Abnormal rhythms (arrhythmias).
- Cardiogenic shock – multiple organs can start to fail because the heart is not able to adequately supply them with blood.
- Cardiac rupture – after the above two complications, both of which can lead to death, this is the commonest cause of fatality. It occurs in 10 per cent of cases, usually between days five to ten as the damaged heart muscle is healing. Rupture takes place through this weakened muscle.
- Heart failure – the heart attack may have weakened the heart and compromised its ability to function properly as a pump. This may need ongoing medication.
- Rupture of papillary muscles – these are muscles inside the heart which operate the heart valves. This can lead to incompetence of the valve and rapid heart failure.
- Pericarditis – inflammation of the sac that contains the heart. This occurs 24 to 72 hours after the event and causes further tight chest pain. It occurs in 20 per cent of patients. It is usually self-limiting, meaning that it settles spontaneously.

## Risk factors for heart disease

There are several factors that put people at high risk of developing acute coronary syndrome and therefore of suffering angina or a heart attack:

- Smoking
- High blood pressure
- Obesity and being overweight
- Raised cholesterol
- Inactivity and sedentary lifestyle

- Poor diet with too much animal fat
- Diabetes (although this is currently under dispute unless the patient also has high blood pressure)
- Previous family history
- Ethnic group (certain groups are more at risk, e.g. British Asians)

## Hardening of the arteries

The medical term for this underlying problem is arteriosclerosis. It is commonly referred to as hardening of the arteries.

As mentioned earlier, blood vessels have a lining of a single layer of epithelial cells. As long as this epithelial lining is intact, then the blood flows smoothly.

If you think of arteries as being like rivers, then you can get an idea of the way arteriosclerosis will build up. It is a bit like the silting up of a river. At bends in the blood vessels, there will be a tendency for silting to take place. It does not just result in a deposit like sand, but in the build-up of what's called *atheroma plaque*.

### What happens next

The plaque is rather like a fatty streak in the vessel wall. Fat molecules get absorbed through the epithelial lining to form a swelling in the vessel wall. Calcium and other minerals may also get trapped in it and fibrous tissue forms to create a hard lumpiness that will narrow the calibre of the vessel and also make it harder and less flexible.

Lots of plaques can develop along the course of an artery, the net effect being to narrow it along a significant length, thereby reducing the flow of blood through it. If this happens in the coronary arteries which supply the heart, then angina may be the result.

### Thrombosis

As long as the integrity of the epithelial lining is maintained, then the blood will flow. However, if that layer is disrupted by the rupture of a plaque, then messenger chemicals will alert blood cells, which will move to the area to form a clot to seal off the damaged part of the vessel. Platelets will accumulate and a fibrous structure like a spider's web will be formed to catch more cells to help to seal the damage. This is called a *thrombus*. The process of thrombus formation is called *thrombosis*.

If the coronary artery is very narrow and the thrombus becomes big enough to block off the flow of blood, then a heart attack is likely. The part of the heart which is supplied by that artery will die.

## Aspirin's role in reducing thrombosis

From what we know about the way that aspirin works, it seems that it helps to reduce the risk of thrombosis by two main mechanisms:

1. It directly reduces inflammation in the blood vessel wall, by blocking the COX-2 enzyme.
2. It also blocks the COX-1 enzyme, which prevents thromboxane from being produced (see page 52). This reduces platelet stickiness and clumping, so will reduce the tendency for the clot to form. The effect will last for the entire 7–9-day lifetime of the individual platelet.

## Different types of heart attack

Heart attacks occur when a blockage in a coronary artery stops oxygenated blood from reaching the heart. They are classified according to which part of the heart is affected, which can usually be diagnosed by ECG. The main areas for heart attacks are:

* The front of the heart. A heart attack located here is called an 'anterior infarct'. This type of heart attack results from blockage of the left coronary artery. This tends to affect the left ventricle, which supplies blood to the whole of the body, except the lungs. These tend to be 'large' heart attacks and are the most dangerous.
* The bottom of the heart (inferior infarct). This is caused by a thrombosis in one of the branches of the right coronary artery. They are usually smaller heart attacks.
* Behind the heart (posterior infarct). These are not always apparent and can be surprisingly hard to diagnose sometimes.

## Investigation of a suspected heart attack

This must be done as quickly as possible, since mortality is greatest soon after a heart attack.

* ECG or electrocardiogram – this measures the electrical activity of the heart. The part of the heart affected will be electrically neutral (as dead tissue will not conduct the electrical activity) so its position will be located on the ECG.
* Blood tests for cardiac enzymes, which are leached into the blood from the dead tissue, will show a rise in their levels. Other blood chemicals will also show a raised level.
* Nuclear imaging – this is a very sophisticated test using nuclear isotopes that will accumulate in the heart tissue and which are quickly cleared from the body. They will determine precisely an area of heart damage.

- Stress test – this is often done after a heart attack before one leaves hospital to determine how well the heart is functioning. If the stress test indicates a need for it, a coronary angiogram (see below) may be arranged.
- Coronary angiography – injecting a dye into the arterial system, which will outline the coronary arteries on a special X-ray. This has to be done in a special X-ray catheter laboratory. It will show blockages that may be improved by putting in a stent to keep them open, or which may need to be repaired in a heart bypass operation.
- Echocardiogram – may also be done to examine the way that the heart is functioning.

## Immediate treatment of a heart attack

The main aim of treatment is to break up a thrombus or clot, to reduce platelet stickiness and clumping, and stop platelets adhering to the damaged plaque (which only increases the size of thrombus, further narrowing the arteries). If this can be done, then further *myocardial ischaemia* (incidents of lack of oxygen to the heart) will be reduced or minimized.

- **Aspirin is the drug of choice in treating heart attacks** (assuming no contraindications, i.e. a medical history which prevents the prescribing of aspirin, such as a haemorrhagic stroke or other haemorrhagic condition, stomach ulcer history, asthma or allergy). GPs all tend to carry this in their bags. A dose of 300mg is given by mouth straight away.
- Other antiplatelet drugs like clopidogrel may be given in hospital.
- Thrombolytic or clot-busting drugs like streptokinase may be given in hospital.

- Other drugs to deal with pain and treat heart failure may be given.

# KEY RESEARCH STUDIES

## Aspirin and secondary heart attack prevention

The first research on heart attack prevention was done on *secondary prevention*. It was known that men were twenty times more likely to have a heart attack if they had already had one. It was therefore important to find out whether a second heart attack could be prevented.

### The first positive research

In the 1970s, the MRC Epidemiology Unit in South Wales began conducting trials on aspirin. They studied a group of men who had *already* had a heart attack and performed a randomized trial in which they were either given a single daily dose of aspirin or a placebo. The trial was published in the *British Medical Journal* in 1974.[9]

- 1,239 men were included.
- A total mortality reduction of 12 per cent was found after six months.
- A total mortality reduction of 24 per cent was found after twelve months.

The problem with this trial was that it was just not large enough. Although the reduction of 24 per cent seems huge, there were not enough men in the trial to give a statistically conclusive result.

There were several more trials on aspirin performed by

different groups over the following years, but they all suffered from insufficient numbers in each trial.

## The first major trial

In 1988, a large international trial was published in *The Lancet*.[10] This was ISIS-2 or the Second International Study of Infarct Survival. It was to have a major impact on clinical practice, for it showed that both aspirin and streptokinase could effect a marked improvement in survival after a heart attack.

The trial was a factorial evaluation of low dose aspirin (160mg), an antiplatelet agent, and streptokinase, a thrombolytic (clot-busting) agent. The study involved 17,187 patients admitted to 417 hospitals with a median time of 5 hours from the onset of symptoms. The patients were randomized with placebo control, so they would receive:

- A one-hour i.v. infusion of 1.5 MU of streptokinase
- One month of 160mg/day enteric-coated aspirin
- Both of the above
- None of the above

The trial concluded that each agent on its own was found to have lowered vascular mortality within the next 35 days by about 25 per cent. However, very significantly, **the death rate was reduced by 42 per cent in the people who received both agents**.

## Independent studies

In the meantime, several independent, smaller scale studies on aspirin's role in preventing a second heart attack were being carried out. In order to utilize the findings of these smaller studies, a meta-analysis was conducted. A meta-analysis is a means of combining the findings from good quality independent trials, giving due weight to their results to assess a treatment effect.

A meta-analysis in 1988 of several trials was highly suggestive of the benefit of low dose aspirin's ability to prevent a second non-fatal heart attack.[11]

## Results in the 1990s

In 1994, the Antithrombotic Trialists' Collaboration performed a meta-analysis on 145 randomized trials of antiplatelet agents, mainly aspirin, against controlled groups. In addition, 29 randomized comparisons between different antiplatelet regimens were included.[12] Effectively, the study featured 70,000 high-risk patients, many of whom had previously had a heart attack.

They found:

* A reduction of one third in non-fatal heart attacks.
* A reduction in strokes by one third.
* A reduction in other vascular deaths by one third.
* Most trials lasted 2–3 years. There seemed to be further reductions after 2–3 years, implying that with longer use, there might be greater improvement.
* Those people at low risk seemed to have a reduced risk of a non-fatal heart attack by one third. This would *imply* a primary prevention of a first heart attack. Clearly, this was a highly important finding.

## Conclusions

The evidence was overwhelming:

* **In people who had a previous major event, such as a heart attack, low dose aspirin could reduce the risk of having a further heart attack or an ischaemic stroke.**

- There was not yet firm evidence of the benefit of aspirin or other antiplatelet drugs in *primary* prevention. More research was needed.

## Aspirin and primary heart attack prevention

### The first study

In 2002, The Antithrombotic Trialists' Collaboration did another meta-analysis.[13] This included both primary and secondary prevention trials of antithrombotic agents, mainly aspirin.

They analysed 287 trials involving over 135,000 patients in comparisons of various antiplatelet agents against placebo or dummy treatment. They also included a further 77,000 patients in comparisons between different active antiplatelet drugs.

- There was a reduction of *any* serious vascular event by about a quarter.
- There was a non-fatal heart attack reduction of one third.
- There was a non-fatal stroke reduction by a quarter.
- There was a reduction in vascular mortality by one sixth.
- The absolute benefit substantially outweighed the risks of a bleed.
- Aspirin was the most widely used antiplatelet drug.

They concluded that aspirin is an effective drug for both primary and secondary prevention in patients at high risk of having a heart attack or a non-haemorrhagic stroke.

## High and low risk patients

The question that was already being asked by many researchers, and which the Antithrombotic Trialists' Collaboration in 1994 posed, was whether aspirin had a place in primary prevention of heart attacks. That is, preventing a first ever event.

As we have just seen, the 2002 Antithrombotic Trialists' Collaboration confirmed that it *did* have a place in primary prevention in patients at *high* risk of having a heart attack or a stroke.

But should people who have no reason to believe they might have a heart attack or stroke take a low dose aspirin each day, 'just in case'?

# The six main trials on primary prevention

There have been six main trials that have looked at aspirin's ability to prevent a primary major event, be that a heart attack or a stroke.

### Trial 1: British Doctors' Trial (BDT)

This included 5,139 healthy doctors who were either given full dose aspirin or no aspirin. The results were published in 1988.

- Total mortality was reduced by 10 per cent in the aspirin group.
- There was no significant reduction in heart attack or stroke.
- There was a slight reduction in mini-strokes (known as transient cerebral ischaemic attacks, or TIAs).

It was felt that the results were not statistically significant since the sample was small and 30 per cent of the aspirin group stopped taking it.

## Trial 2: The Physicians' Health Study (PHS)

This was a randomized factorial designed trial (see glossary) involving 22,071 American physicians. They received alternate day aspirin and beta-carotene to determine whether there was a reduction in the incidence of cancer. Although the study was not intended to examine the effects of aspirin on the heart, the researchers nevertheless noted these results, which were published in 1989.[14]

- There was a 44 per cent reduction in first non-fatal heart attack.
- There was an 18 per cent reduction in non-fatal stroke.
- There was an 18 per cent reduction in fatal events.

## Trial 3: Hypertension Optimal Treatment Study (HOT)

This study looked at the effect of aspirin on treatments used to bring down high blood pressure. Patients were randomized with low dose aspirin so that 9,399 received aspirin and a similar number received a placebo. They also all received their regular treatment for high blood pressure.

The results were published in 1998.[15] Aspirin reduced all heart attacks, both fatal and non-fatal, by 36 per cent.

## Trial 4: Thrombosis Prevention Trial (TPT)

This included 5,499 men aged 49–65 at entry to the trial, all calculated to be at high risk of having a major heart event or a stroke. They were recruited from 108 general practices, all of which were part of the Medical Research Council's GP

Research Framework. A factorial design was used, so that men were randomized to receive a combination of either active aspirin and active warfarin; active aspirin and placebo warfarin; placebo aspirin and active warfarin; or double placebo. When given, aspirin and warfarin were both given in low dose.

The results were published in *The Lancet* in 1998.[16] The researchers were investigating the impact of the drugs on all types of heart disease caused by blockages in the circulatory system (known as ischaemic heart disease, or IHD), which was defined as the sum of coronary death and fatal and non-fatal heart attacks.

- The main effect of warfarin was a reduction in all IHD of 21 per cent, due to a 39 per cent reduction in fatal events, so that warfarin reduced the death rate from *all* causes by 17 per cent.
- The main effect of aspirin was a reduction in IHD of 20 per cent, due to a reduction of 32 per cent of non-fatal events.
- The combination of both drugs reduced all IHD by 34 per cent compared to placebo.

Conclusions:

- This study added to the evidence that aspirin reduces non-fatal IHD.
- Warfarin reduced all IHD mainly because of a reduction in fatal events.
- Combined aspirin and warfarin seemed more effective in the reduction of IHD than either agent on its own.

### Trial 5: The Primary Prevention Project (PPP)

This was another factorial designed trial in which patients were given low dose aspirin (100mg) in enteric-coated form and/or vitamin E, in addition to other lifestyle advice and treatment of risk factors to see whether it could reduce the risk of a major event in the brain or heart (i.e. a stroke or heart attack).

There were 4,495 patients included, both males and females of 50 years and over, all of whom had at least one risk factor for a heart attack (diabetes, raised cholesterol, old age, obesity, high blood pressure or a family history of premature heart attacks).

The trial was stopped prematurely owing to results shown in the TPT and HOT trials. The results were published in 2001.[17]

- There was a 44 per cent reduction in relative risk of all cardiovascular events, including heart attack, sudden death and non-fatal stroke.
- Low dose aspirin was effective in both males and females.
- Vitamin E showed no effect on outcome.

### Trial 6: The Women's Health Study (WHS)

In this double-blind placebo-controlled study, apparently healthy women aged 45 and over at entry to the study were given low dose aspirin on alternate days either with vitamin E or placebo. The trial included almost 40,000 women who were followed up for ten years. The results were published in 2005.[18]

- There was a 17 per cent reduction in the risk of having a stroke.
- There was a 19 per cent reduction in non-fatal stroke.
- There was a 22 per cent reduction in the risk of having a mini-stroke.
- In women over the age of 65, there was a 26 per cent reduction in cardiovascular events.
- There did not seem to be a benefit in regards to heart attacks.

## The latest picture

In 2009, the Antithrombotic Trialists' Collaboration[19] performed another meta-analysis of the six primary prevention trials that we have just run through (95,000 people who were at low average risk of having a major event), and in addition sixteen secondary prevention trials (17,000 people at high risk of an event).

In the primary prevention trials:

- Aspirin showed an average 12 per cent reduction in serious vascular events – mainly due to a reduction in heart attacks.
- No significant reduction in the incidence of strokes was shown.
- Aspirin increased the risk of major gastrointestinal (stomach) and extracranial (brain) bleeds.

In the secondary prevention trials:

- Aspirin showed a greater reduction in serious vascular events.
- There was a reduction in the incidence of strokes of 20 per cent.

In both primary and secondary prevention trials:

- The proportional reductions seen were the same for males and females.

Conclusions:

- Although there is certainly evidence of the benefit of taking aspirin for those people who have *definite* occlusive disease (evidence of narrowing of the arteries), and for those who are at high risk of having a heart attack or a stroke, the same

evidence is *not* there for people at low risk with no evidence of disease.
- While there may be a slight reduction in the risk of major events for such low-risk patients, this would have to be balanced against the risk of having a major bleed.

### CHAPTER SUMMARY

We can draw three general conclusions about the use of aspirin in preventing heart disease:

1. Aspirin is an effective drug for both primary and secondary prevention in patients at high risk of having an event (see page 78 for a list of risk factors to see if you may fall into this high-risk category). In some studies, taking aspirin reduced the likelihood of a cardiovascular problem (heart disease, heart attack or stroke) for such patients by as much as **44 per cent**.
2. In patients who had already suffered a major event, such as a heart attack or an ischaemic stroke, daily low dose aspirin could significantly reduce the risk of having a further heart attack or a further ischaemic stroke by as much as **33 per cent**. The risks of suffering from a side effect of aspirin (such as a bleed) are *less* than the risks of non-treatment. Therefore, aspirin use is recommended for patients who have previously suffered a heart attack or ischaemic stroke in order to prevent a secondary event (assuming their medical history allows them to receive aspirin, of course).
3. Aspirin is of uncertain benefit in reducing the risk of having a cardiovascular event in people who are only at low risk. Any benefit would have to be balanced against the risk of suffering side effects. However, aspirin's benefits against other conditions, like cancer, may need to be taken into consideration

when one discusses with one's doctor whether or not to take it. Its overall effect on several conditions may persuade you to take it on a regular basis as a preventative measure against a variety of diseases, regardless of the risk of possible side effects – but this is a decision for you and your doctor.

# STROKES 7

Although we have mentioned strokes as a major cardiovascular event in the last chapter, they merit some special consideration.

## Some stroke statistics

* The brain receives 25 per cent of the body's oxygen, but it cannot store it.
* If the blood supply to part of the brain is cut off, brain cells start to die very quickly.
* The World Health Organization estimates that there were 1.4 million deaths from strokes in Europe in 1999.
* According to the World Stroke Organization, somewhere in the world someone dies from a stroke every six seconds
* According to the World Stroke Organization, one person in six is liable to have a stroke in their lifetime.
* There are approximately 110,000 first strokes in the UK per year.
* There are approximately 30,000 recurrent strokes in the UK per year.
* Strokes are the third commonest cause of death (11 per cent of deaths in England and Wales).
* Strokes are the commonest cause of long-term disability in the UK.
* There are 500,000 stroke victims living in the community in the UK.

## Types of stroke

A cerebrovascular accident or a stroke is the name given to brain attack in which an area of the brain is deprived of its blood supply. As a result, brain cells will start to die off and others may be left damaged.

Most strokes happen when a blood clot blocks off an artery in the brain. This is called an *ischaemic stroke*.

There are several types of ischaemic stroke:

- Transient Ischaemic Attack (TIA) – this is a mini-stroke that lasts less than 24 hours. The blockage is only transient and normal flow is re-established by the body. It must be treated seriously, however, since it may be a warning of a serious major stroke.
- Cerebral thrombosis – this is the formation of a blood clot in one of the cerebral arteries that is already narrowed and partially furred up.
- Cerebral embolism – this is a stroke due to a clot that has arisen in another part of the body being hurtled into the cerebral circulation and lodging in a narrowed artery. The likeliest cause is an irregular heartbeat, such as atrial fibrillation (see page 76).

Another dangerous type of stroke is the *haemorrhagic stroke*. This occurs when a blood vessel in the brain bursts and blood seeps into the brain tissue, causing damage. If the blood flow does not stop, this can be rapidly fatal.

## Symptoms of a stroke

These are variable, depending on which part of the brain has been affected.

Common symptoms are:

- Weakness of one side of the face, possibly with drooping lip
- Weakness or paralysis of one side of the body
- Slurred or difficult speech
- Difficulty swallowing
- Partial loss of vision or visual difficulty
- Headache
- Confusion
- Involuntary evacuation of bowel or bladder
- Diminishing consciousness or loss of consciousness

## Dr Thomas Willis

In the last chapter we mentioned William Harvey, who discovered how the circulation of the blood worked.

Contemporary with him was Dr Thomas Willis (1621–75), another royal physician who fought on the royalist side during the English Civil War. Like Harvey, he was an anatomist who was deeply interested in the blood supply of the body.

Willis published several books in the 1660s, the most significant being a work about the brain. In it, he described the circle of blood vessels at the base of the brain, which is formed from the major arteries travelling up the front of the neck as well as the ones from the back. These arteries join together to produce an arterial circle, from which branches supply blood to the various areas of the brain. This is called the Circle of Willis. A blockage in the Circle of Willis or in any of its branches will result in a stroke.

## Treatment of a stroke

Hospitalization is important in order to diagnose the type of stroke.

- Ischaemic strokes may receive clot-busting, thrombolytic agents like streptokinase and antiplatelet agents like aspirin.
- Haemorrhagic strokes **MUST NOT** receive thrombolytic agents or aspirin, which could make matters worse. This advice continues even after the stroke is over, so that any patient who has ever had a haemorrhagic stroke should *never* again receive aspirin – for life.

There would also be treatment of underlying conditions.

## Risk factors for having a stroke

By and large, these are the same as for a heart attack (see page 78), but with emphasis on the following:

- Irregular heartbeat, especially atrial fibrillation. Between 2 to 4 per cent of people with atrial fibrillation without a history of TIA or of stroke *will* have a major stroke within a year
- Previous history of TIA or stroke
- High blood pressure
- Smoking
- Diabetes (although this is currently under dispute unless the patient also has high blood pressure)
- Drinking – anything above the adult recommended limits of 28 units per week for a man and 21 units per week for a woman. People who drink too much are also at risk of liver disease and dementia

## Can aspirin prevent strokes?

Various studies have been conducted about this important question. The key studies are set out below, together with their results.

## The 1977 study

The first positive study that showed aspirin *was* protective against strokes was published in 1977. This was a small double-blind controlled trial by Fields et al. on aspirin in cerebral ischemia (incidents of lack of blood flow to the brain).[20] It included 178 patients who had a history of TIAs (mini-strokes).

- Started in 1972 and ran for 37 months.
- Patients randomly received either aspirin or placebo.
- The measurable end points of the trial were subsequent TIA, death, cerebral or retinal infarction (the death of parts of the tissue in the brain or eye, usually due to blocked arteries).

Results:

- At six months of follow-up, there was a significant reduction in incidence of TIAs, death, cerebral and retinal infarctions.
- The most impressive results occurred when there was a history of repeated TIAs.

## The UK-TIA Trial

This was a trial that ran from 1979 to 1985, involving 2,435 patients with a history of TIA.[21]

- They were randomized to receive either 600mg aspirin twice a day, or 300mg daily, or placebo.
- There was no difference in efficacy between the 300mg aspirin or 1200mg aspirin groups – but the 1200mg group had more gastric side effects.
- There was no difference between males and females.

The researchers found that odds of suffering a stroke, heart attack or death were 15 per cent lower in the combined aspirin groups than in the placebo group.

### The International Stroke Trial

This was a large study[22], published in 1997, of 19,435 patients who had had an ischaemic stroke. They were randomized to receive either aspirin or heparin (an anticoagulant – anti-clotting agent – given by injection) for 14 days starting immediately after the stroke.

At six months follow-up, aspirin was associated with a reduced incidence of death or subsequent dependency* in 13 events per 1,000 patients. Heparin showed no effect.

### The Chinese Acute Stroke Trial

This randomized placebo-controlled trial followed up 20,000 patients with an acute ischaemic stroke.[23] Antithrombotic (anti-clotting) therapy was given for four weeks. Aspirin was associated with a 12 per cent reduction of in-hospital death or non-fatal stroke at four weeks. It also reduced death or dependency at discharge by 11.4 events per 1,000 patients.

## AF and strokes

Everyone with atrial fibrillation (or AF – see page 76) is at increased risk of having a stroke. In short, AF is the irregular beating of the heart, which makes clot formation within the heart likely. These clots can then enter the bloodstream and travel to the brain, causing a stroke.

---

* By 'dependency', I mean a reduced capability to care for oneself following a stroke, so that dependency on a carer for basic needs is a result.

The National Institute for Health and Clinical Excellence, NICE, advises that doctors divide people with atrial fibrillation into three grades of risk:

1. **High risk** – 6–12 in a 100 chance of having a stroke in the next 12 months
   - Aged more than 75 years
   - Previous stroke
   - Heart valve problem
   - Existing heart failure

2. **Moderate risk** – 3–5 in a 100 chance of having a stroke in the next 12 months
   - Aged 65 years or older
   - Any age up to 75 years with one of the following – high blood pressure, diabetes, heart disease or peripheral arterial disease (see page 104)

3. **Low risk** – 1–2 in a 100 chance of having a stroke in the next 12 months
   - Aged younger than 65 years with no other risk factors

---

### AF

- 50,000 new cases each year.
- 1 in 200 people aged 50–60 years have atrial fibrillation.
- 1 in 10 people over 80 years have atrial fibrillation.

---

## Aspirin and AF

Aspirin is just one way of treating AF (other methods are explained below), but it is proven to be effective. According to the current NICE recommendations:

- In patients with atrial fibrillation classified at *low risk* of a stroke, aspirin in a daily dose of 75mg to 300mg should be given, assuming no contraindications.
- In patients with atrial fibrillation classified at *moderate risk* of a stroke, a daily dose of 75mg to 300mg of aspirin should be given *or* anticoagulation (using drugs such as warfarin) should be considered.
- In patients with atrial fibrillation classified at *high risk* of a stroke, warfarin should be given to maintain blood-controlled anticoagulation, provided there is no contraindication. If there is a contraindication, then aspirin should be considered, provided there are no contraindications to it.

## Treatment of AF

There are four ways of treating AF:

- Reduce the heart rate: with drugs like beta-blockers.
- Reduce the rhythm:
    1. With cardioversion in a few cases. This is an electric shock to jolt the heart back into a normal rhythm.
    2. With anti-arrhythmic drugs.
- Thinning the blood:
    1. Anticoagulation with warfarin – to prevent blood clots being formed by the butter-churn action of the fibrillating atria. This is 80 per cent likely to prevent clots.
    
    OR
    
    2. Antiplatelet drugs like aspirin, if the patient cannot be anticoagulated. This is 20 per cent likely to prevent clots.
- Other treatments: involving treatment of thyroid problem, or surgery for heart valve problem, or treatment of high blood pressure.

## The BAFTA Study

Over the years, there had been seven trials on warfarin and aspirin in the prevention of strokes. They had shown that warfarin was effective in 80 per cent of cases and aspirin in 20 per cent. Yet it had not been determined whether the benefit in elderly patients outweighed the potential risk of using anticoagulants.

The risk is of producing a bleed in the brain or in the stomach. The fact that patients taking warfarin have to have regular blood tests to check that the blood is not too thin also has to be taken into account, as this can be distressing and inconvenient for some patients.

In 2007, an important study, the Birmingham Atrial Fibrillation Treatment of the Aged Study, was carried out in over 200 general practices in the UK to compare the use of aspirin and warfarin in the treatment of atrial fibrillation in patients over the age of 75 years in order to prevent strokes.[24] This is known as the BAFTA study.

- 973 patients over the age of 75 years were recruited and were randomly allocated to receive either warfarin or aspirin.
- There were 24 primary events (strokes and embolism) in the warfarin group.
- There were 48 primary events (strokes and embolism) in the aspirin group.

Conclusions:

- This study data supported the use of anticoagulation therapy for people aged over 75 who have atrial fibrillation, unless there are contraindications or the patient decides that the benefits are not worth the inconvenience (i.e. of having to have regular blood tests).
- If they do not feel that they wish to take anticoagulation drugs, then aspirin would offer less, yet some, protection.

# STROKES

**CHAPTER SUMMARY**

Aspirin has been shown to be effective as both an active *and* preventative treatment of strokes. This means it can both prevent strokes, and act as a medicine in the treatment of them if they occur.

*As an active treatment*

- The Royal College of Physicians and the National Institute for Health and Clinical Excellence currently recommend that patients should be given 300mg of aspirin after a stroke, as soon as a haemorrhagic stroke has been excluded.
- Anyone who has had a haemorrhagic stroke should *not* receive aspirin. There would be the risk of producing a further bleed in the brain, which could result in death.

*As a preventative treatment*

- Patients who have had a mini-stroke should take aspirin. Suffering from mini-strokes (TIA) can be a sign that a major event is on the way. Aspirin has been proven to be effective at reducing the chance of stroke, heart attack and death in TIA patients by **15 per cent**. It also reduces the risk of further mini-strokes.
- Patients with atrial fibrillation are at increased risk of having a stroke: between 2 to 4 per cent of people with AF will have a major stroke within a year. Daily low dose aspirin is recommended for AF patients classed at low and moderate risk, and for high-risk patients who are unable to take anticoagulants.
- After experiencing their first non-haemorrhagic stroke, patients should be prescribed 50–300mg aspirin daily indefinitely, in order to prevent further events.

# 8. ARTERIES, VEINS AND ASPIRIN IN PREGNANCY

We now need to consider the blood supply to the rest of the body. It can get complicated, so we shall first consider problems with the arterial system (which takes oxygenated blood to the tissues), then with the venous system (which returns deoxygenated blood to the heart).

It has always been thought that aspirin could help both types of problem. But as we shall see, research shows that this is not the case.

## ARTERIES

### Peripheral arterial disease

Peripheral arterial disease means disease of the arterial system to the limbs. For practical purposes, it refers to the narrowing of the blood supply (also known as occlusive disease) to the lower limbs.

The pathology is exactly the same as with the heart disease we have already discussed on page 79 – it is arteriosclerosis (hardening of the arteries) affecting the arteries of the lower limbs.

- The classic symptom is called *intermittent claudication*. This is pain developing in the calf muscles or sometimes in the buttocks on walking a distance. This distance is variable. Some people only get it on walking a few hundred yards, others as little as thirty yards. Stopping to rest eases the pain.
- Such symptoms should always be investigated.
- If peripheral arterial disease is present, then the individual is likely to have coronary artery disease and cerebrovascular disease. Indeed, half will have a history of either a previous stroke or a heart attack.
- They are therefore at risk of stroke and heart attack.

## Can aspirin help?

Let's look at the research conducted so far. The CAPRIE study, published in 1996, was a randomized, blinded trial of the drug clopidogrel versus aspirin in patients at risk of an ischaemic stroke (a stroke caused by lack of blood flow to the brain).[25] It was a secondary prevention trial with 19,158 patients. The study population consisted of three groups, with about 6,300 patients in each sub-group:

1. Those who had had a recent stroke
2. Those who had had a recent heart attack
3. Those with symptomatic peripheral arterial disease

Clopidogrel was found to be slightly more effective than aspirin in protecting against a second stroke, a second heart attack or death. (Interestingly, despite the result of this trial, aspirin is still considered to be the mainstay of treatment and clopidogrel is reserved for patients who cannot tolerate aspirin. This could be due to the fact that aspirin is considerably cheaper.)

However, the study found that aspirin does *not* seem to have any effect on people whose main problem is their peripheral arterial disease. Nonetheless, the conclusion of the trial was that patients with peripheral arterial disease should be prescribed either clopidogrel or aspirin in a dose of 75mg to 300mg daily. Although this may seem difficult to evaluate, the point is that at least half the people who have peripheral arterial disease will also have coronary or cerebral vascular disease (i.e. the same arterial problem near their heart or brain), so they *will* benefit from aspirin's ability to reduce their risk of a serious event. For this reason, aspirin is seen to be a sensible drug to take if you have peripheral arterial disease, provided there are no contraindications.

## ASPIRIN IN PREGNANCY

It would seem appropriate to consider this subject at this point, since aspirin has been proven to assist with a handful of potential problems in pregnancy that are directly related to the arteries.

It is important to note that, in general, aspirin is *not* recommended during pregnancy. This is because any drug taken as an embryo is developing could have an adverse effect on that development at a critical point, possibly resulting in abnormalities.

### Miscarriage

There is also a theoretical risk of provoking a bleed underneath the placenta, which could result in a miscarriage.

Two Danish studies published in the *British Medical Journal* (*BMJ*) in 2001 looked at the effects of taking aspirin and other NSAIDs before and during pregnancy.[26] The first study involved 1,462 pregnant women who had taken aspirin or other NSAIDs in the period of 30 days before conception until birth and 17,259 pregnant women who had not taken any drugs. The second study compared 4,268 women who had a miscarriage (68 of whom had taken aspirin or NSAIDs) and 29,750 women who had live births.

The researchers found that there seemed to be an association between the taking of the drugs and miscarriage. The greatest association was with those who had taken the drug a week before the miscarriage.

They concluded that there seemed to be an association with taking the drug and miscarriage, but they were unable to say that taking the drug caused a miscarriage. Nonetheless, the general guidance issued to women is as follows:

- Aspirin is not recommended for routine use by pregnant women.
- Aspirin should not be taken by any woman attempting to conceive.

## High blood pressure

The condition of high blood pressure (hypertension) in pregnancy, however, provides special cases when it may be appropriate to take aspirin prescribed by a doctor:

- Intrauterine growth retardation (IUGR)
- Pre-eclampsia

Both of these are caused by problems in the small arteries in the placenta. In the first, the developing baby's growth is compromised and the pregnancy is at risk. In the second, the blood pressure may rise dangerously high. It affects between 5 and 8 per cent of pregnancies. In the UK, severe cases cause the deaths of up to ten women a year and up to 1,000 babies.

Women with the following are at high risk of hypertensive disorders in pregnancy:

- Hypertensive disease during a previous pregnancy
- Chronic kidney disease
- Autoimmune disease such as systemic lupus erythematosis, or antiphospholipid syndrome
- Type 1 or type 2 diabetes
- Chronic hypertension

## What the studies show

In 1998, a randomized trial of low dose aspirin for the prevention and treatment of pre-eclampsia – the CLASP trial – was published in *The Lancet*.[27]

- 9,364 women were included.
- 74 per cent were entered to see if aspirin would prevent pre-eclampsia.
- 12 per cent were entered to see if aspirin would prevent IUGR.
- 12 per cent were entered for treatment of pre-eclampsia.
- 3 per cent were entered for treatment of IUGR.
- They were given either 60mg of aspirin or a placebo.

The researchers found:

- Aspirin use was associated with a reduction of 12 per cent in pre-eclampsia.
- There was no significant effect on the incidence of IUGR, stillbirth and neonatal death.
- There was a significant trend towards greater reduction of pre-eclampsia the more pre-term the delivery.
- There was no increase in placental haemorrhages in the aspirin group.
- There was a slight increase in the need for blood transfusion after birth.

Conclusions:

- They concluded that aspirin was generally safe for mother and baby in the trial with no increased risk in bleeding.
- They did not feel, however, that they were justified in recommending low dose aspirin to *all* women at increased risk of IUGR or of pre-eclampsia as a preventative measure.
- They did say that low dose aspirin may be deemed appropriate in women who would be liable to early-onset pre-eclampsia severe enough to need very pre-term delivery.

Meanwhile, in 2007, a meta-analysis was made of data on 32,217 women and their 32,819 babies, who had been recruited into 31 trials.[28] They showed that the risk of developing pre-eclampsia, delivering before 34 weeks of pregnancy and of having a pregnancy with a severely poor outcome was reduced by 10 per cent in women who took either aspirin or other antiplatelet agents.

---

### THE NICE GUIDELINES

The current NICE guidelines recommend that women at high risk of pre-eclampsia should take 75mg of aspirin daily, **under the care of their doctor**, from 12 weeks until the birth of their baby.

Under no circumstances should pregnant women self-medicate with aspirin.

# VEINS

It would seem logical to think that if aspirin has a beneficial effect on problems of the arteries, it would also be useful in problems with the veins.

There is a big difference between arteries and veins, however. Veins have valves in them. Not just that, but they are one-way valves. Their purpose is to prevent blood from flowing backwards between heartbeats, when the heart is filling up and the circulation is not being driven onwards by the force of the pump.

## Varicose veins

The number of valves that people have per segment of vein varies from person to person. If you are fortunate and have many, then you are less liable to suffer from varicose veins. This is because each valve has to support the weight of the column of blood above it all the way up to the next valve. If you have lots of valves, then the column that each valve has to support is quite short and the weight of blood will not be too heavy. It will easily withstand the pressure.

On the other hand, if the column of blood is long and heavy, there will be pressure on that valve between every heartbeat. It may become incompetent and allow blood to leak backwards. This causes a bulge around the valve. Eventually, the whole vein will bulge. That is, the vein will start to become varicose.

Varicose veins can occur in many parts of the body, the most common sites being the lower legs and the rectum (when they are called haemorrhoids). They can also occur in the oesophagus (the part of the body which connects the throat to the stomach), particularly when there is liver disease and a condition called portal hypertension (most likely in alcoholism).

Disappointingly for the many sufferers of this condition, there is no evidence that aspirin has any effect whatsoever on varicose veins.

## Blood clots in the veins

Venous thromboembolism (VTE) is the name given to the development of a blood clot forming in the lower limb or pelvic veins. This clot can fragment and produce an embolus, which may be carried to the lungs, where it can lodge in a blood vessel – with potentially catastrophic results. This is called a pulmonary embolism.

- A deep-vein thrombosis (DVT) is the name for a thrombus or clot that forms in one of these veins of the lower limb, most often in a vein in the calf.
- A clot that fragments off to float in the blood is called an embolus.
- A pulmonary embolism (PE) is the name for a loose clot or embolus from a DVT that lodges in a lung vessel.
- 20 per cent of untreated DVTs will develop a PE.
- In the UK, 25,000 people die each year from VTE: a greater number than the combined figures of deaths due to breast cancer, accidents and AIDS.
- Post-thrombotic syndrome is a complication after a DVT. The leg may stay swollen with fluid, called oedema. Leg ulceration may be the result.

### Virchow's triad

The German physician Rudolph Virchow (1821–1902) was the first person to deduce the link between a DVT and a pulmonary embolism. He also formulated a triad of conditions that make venous thrombus formation more likely:

- Damage to the inner lining of the vein
- Venous stasis (from immobility – thus why it is sensible to take precautions against developing DVT when sitting still for long periods of time, such as on a long-haul flight. See page 114 for more detail on this common concern)
- Abnormality of the clotting mechanism

### Risk factors for DVT

- Previous history of thromboembolism
- Conditions that cause increased coagulability of the blood (making it thicker and stickier), e.g. various blood disorders and cancer (diagnosed or unknown)
- Factor V Leiden gene.* About 5 per cent of the population have this gene, which predisposes people to a fivefold risk of having a blood clot
- Heart failure
- Increasing age
- Immobility – from stroke, bed-ridden state, plaster casts
- Trauma to blood vessels
- Pregnancy
- Hormone treatments, including the oral contraceptive pill
- Dehydration

## Can aspirin prevent DVT?

Some studies in the past have suggested a benefit from taking aspirin as a preventive measure against the development of DVT. However, recent research does not seem to back up this earlier work.

---

* The presence of the Factor V Leiden gene can be detected by blood test. It does not need treatment unless the blood starts to clot.

## Post-operative DVT

Much research has focused on aspirin's potential to prevent post-operative DVT. One such study was published in 1977 by Harris et al.[29] It was a prospective double-blind study of the use of aspirin as a preventative drug in patients over the age of 40 years who had undergone hip replacement surgery. Those who received aspirin took 600mg twice a day. The researchers found:

- VTE developed in 11 of 44 patients receiving aspirin.
- VTE developed in 23 of 55 patients receiving placebo.
- There was a significantly greater protection for men than women.

Much of the subsequent work that has been done on prevention of DVT post-op has focused on patients receiving total hip replacement or total knee replacement, both of which obviously will result in immobility with the risk of venous stasis, and trauma to blood vessels.

A working party of experts assessed the use of various strategies in the prevention of VTE in hospitalized patients and reported to the UK Chief Medical Officer in 2007.[30] They did *not* recommend the routine use of aspirin as a preventative agent in hospitalized medical or surgical patients. Having said that, some reduction in VTE has been noted following the taking of aspirin, but it has been deemed insufficient by the National Clinical Guidance Centre to recommend it as a prophylactic (preventative agent) for VTE prevention.[31]

## Conclusions

- Aspirin is not currently recommended as a preventative agent for post-operative DVT. Although aspirin has been noted to produce some reduction in VTE, experts

currently deem it insufficient to warrant a recommendation for use.
- Anticoagulants have been found of more benefit in the prevention of VTE.

## The question of travel

This is an important topic, since long-distance journeys have become a normal part of life in developed countries. The immobility that results on aeroplanes, in cars and on trains, together with the pressure of seats on the muscles of the buttocks and behind the knees for long periods, has been seen as a risk factor for the development of DVTs.

In addition, there has been a suggestion that the reduced pressure in air cabins on aeroplanes may in some way be enough to trigger the coagulation mechanism in some people. However, recent research with healthy volunteers sitting in a hypobaric chamber (a chamber which has reduced pressure to simulate air cabin pressure) did *not* find that it triggered clot formation. Whether this could be different in people who have a higher risk is still not known.

---

### ECONOMY CLASS SYNDROME

The association between long-haul flights and DVT was first described in 1954 by a 54-year-old doctor who developed a DVT during a 14-hour flight.

---

Can aspirin lower the risk of DVT on long-haul flights?

It had seemed logical to suppose that aspirin may have a beneficial effect in reducing DVT associated with long-distance travel, since it was known to reduce the risk of blood clots in the arteries.

In 2001, the World Health Organization (WHO) set up the World Health Organization Research into Global Hazards of Travel Project, with the suitable acronym of the WRIGHT Project, evocative of the Wright brothers, the innovators of air travel. Researchers looked at the many factors involved, ranging from body size, position, medical factors, time of travel, etc. Phase 1 was reported in 2007. They found:

- The risk of venous thromboembolism (VTE) doubles when travelling on a flight of more than four hours.
- The absolute risk of VTE even after four hours is low at 1 in 6,000.
- The two commonest manifestations of VTE were DVT and PE (see page 111).
- The risk is increased after a long-haul journey and remains elevated for four weeks.
- Multiple long journeys in a short period increase the risk.

We still do not know whether aspirin will prevent a DVT due to air travel or long journeys. *If* it works, it seems to have a modest benefit. To put this into figures, it is estimated that you would need to treat 17,000 people with aspirin to prevent one DVT.

This figure of 1 in 17,000 is in keeping with a paper published in *Medscape General Medicine* in 2002[32], which calculated the potential benefit of aspirin in reducing the risk of having a DVT, by applying the data for aspirin in preventing DVT in hip fracture patients to the estimated rates of travel-related DVT. They based this on a rate of travel-related DVT of 20 per 100,000 travellers.

In conclusion, aspirin is *not* recommended as a preventive agent for DVT on a long-haul flight or journey for people at *low* risk. Nonetheless, it is an issue that will concern many people. If overly concerned, the individual should discuss it with their doctor. One possibility that might be considered is to take one low dose aspirin (75mg) on the day of a long-haul flight and one low dose aspirin (75mg) daily for three days afterwards.

As ever, the decision to take any drug should first be discussed with your GP.

### CHAPTER SUMMARY

- Aspirin is effective at treating arterial disease and is recommended for patients suffering from peripheral arterial disease (PAD). While it will not necessarily treat or prevent PAD itself, it will reduce patients' risk of having a more serious arterial-related event such as a stroke or a heart attack caused by an arterial blockage. Patients with PAD are at increased risk of having a stroke or heart attack and aspirin will significantly reduce their chance of suffering such a serious event.
- Aspirin is not recommended for routine use by pregnant women. However, for those at risk of developing pre-eclampsia or IUGR, it may be suitable for use as a preventative measure, **but only ever with medical guidance from your doctor**. Some studies have suggested that aspirin reduces the risk of developing pre-eclampsia, having an early delivery or a severely poor outcome by around 10 per cent for women at *high* risk of these conditions.
- Aspirin is currently *not* shown to be an effective treatment for venous problems:
  - It has no effect on varicose veins.
  - It has been noted to produce some reduction in post-operative VTE (see page 113), but experts currently deem it insufficient to warrant a recommendation for use.
  - It is not recommended for use as a preventive agent for DVT on a long-haul flight or journey for people at low risk: studies show it has a 1 in 17,000 chance of being effective for this particular problem.

# ASPIRIN AND DEMENTIA 9

One of the great fears that most people have is that they may lose their mental function and end their days slipping into dementia.

Dementia is the name given to a group of brain disorders that cause a deterioration of intellectual faculties, such as memory, concentration and judgement. There is no impairment of consciousness. It is sometimes accompanied by emotional disturbance and personality changes. The name comes from the Latin *demens*, meaning 'senseless'.

## Some dementia statistics

- Globally, there are more than 35 million people with one or other form of dementia.
- About 25 million people in the UK, or 42 per cent of the population, know a close friend or have a relative with dementia.
- There are 163,000 new cases of dementia in the UK every year.
- Dementia is not a disease of developed countries – 60 per cent of cases of dementia occur in developing countries.

## The different types of dementia

There are several types of dementia recognized these days, including Creutzfeldt-Jakob disease, Korsakoff's psychosis, fronto-temporal dementia and Huntington's chorea, but the most common are:

- Alzheimer's disease: the commonest – accounts for 60–70 per cent of cases of dementia.
- Vascular dementia: the second commonest – 20 per cent.
- Dementia with Lewy bodies – 10 per cent. It has characteristics of both Alzheimer's disease and Parkinson's disease.

## Alzheimer's disease

This is a brain disease that is associated with definite pathological changes in the brain and in brain chemistry.

- Alzheimer's disease affects over 15 million people worldwide.
- Alzheimer's disease affects 465,000 people in the UK.
- The risk of developing Alzheimer's disease doubles every 5 years after the age of 65 years.
- In the UK, there are over 16,000 people under the age of 65 years with Alzheimer's disease.
- There is no known cure for Alzheimer's disease, but there are treatments that may delay the onward progression of the condition.
- Alzheimer's disease is progressive.

### Symptoms

People in the early stages of Alzheimer's disease may simply seem a bit forgetful. It will tend to be the short-term memory that goes first, so that the individual forgets recent events, but will be able to recall events from their childhood with relative clarity.

Gradually, their memory will deteriorate even more, but they may seem to get round it by confabulating. This means by making things up. Indeed, they may even seem to be good at a sort of cocktail party chatter, by just latching onto the other person's conversation and answering questions or talking around things.

Then their cognitive ability starts to deteriorate. They will have difficulty counting, working money out. They may develop mood swings, becoming excessively weepy or irritable. Sometimes their personality will start to change and they may exhibit disinhibited, anti-social or even very bizarre behaviour. They may start to neglect themselves. They may lose a sense of what is dangerous. They may become disorientated and start to wander at night.

### NOT ALL FORGETFULNESS IS ALZHEIMER'S DISEASE

This is an important point. A lot of elderly people develop forgetfulness and experience deterioration in their cognitive thinking ability. It does not mean that they are developing Alzheimer's disease. The condition of Mild Cognitive Impairment (MCI) is not an illness. It is a feature of ageing in some people. Alzheimer's disease, on the other hand, is a disease and is not normal ageing.

Only 10–15 per cent of people who develop MCI will go on to develop Alzheimer's disease.

If someone is showing signs of memory loss or cognitive difficulty, then a mental state examination by their GP should be the first step. If necessary, they can then be referred to a memory clinic for further testing.

### Changes within the brain

In Alzheimer's disease, the brain changes physically in several ways. The net effect of all these changes is to reduce the functioning brain tissue.

The overwhelming characteristic feature found in the brains of people with Alzheimer's disease is *senile plaques*. These are clumps of material formed from degenerated brain cells and a type of protein called beta-amyloid.

It is thought that beta-amyloid can set off a vicious circle. The presence of this substance seems to trigger inflammation. The inflammation then produces more beta-amyloid – and so the cycle continues.

Other changes include the presence of neurofibrillary tangles, shrinking of the brain and enlargement of the ventricles (fluid spaces) in the brain.

### How can aspirin help?

Scientists have discovered that levels of the COX-2 enzyme (which we learned about in chapter 4, see page 49) are found to be raised in certain parts of the brains of people with Alzheimer's disease. It is not conclusive as yet, but this may indicate that prostaglandins have a part to play in the production of beta-amyloid and the build-up of senile plaques in Alzheimer's disease.

This could of course be a mechanism by which aspirin may have a role to play in reducing the risk of the condition, since it blocks the action of the COX-2 enzyme.

## Vascular dementia

This is dementia caused by disturbances arising from the vascular (blood) supply to the brain. There are several types, including:

- Single infarct dementia – when damage occurs from a single stroke.
- Multi-infarct dementia – when damage occurs from a succession of small strokes.
- Small vessel disease dementia – when there is damage to many small blood vessels deep in the brain.

The effects can be similar to Alzheimer's or not as marked. Physical symptoms may be more apparent, as areas of the brain associated with physical functioning may be affected.

## How aspirin may help with dementia

From what we have just discussed, one can see that there are various possible ways in which aspirin might be of value in reducing the risk of developing both Alzheimer's disease and vascular dementia.

1. By blocking the COX-2 enzyme, it might reduce the production of prostaglandins, which *may* have a role in the build-up of beta-amyloid, and the vicious circle that *might* be involved in Alzheimer's disease.
2. By blocking COX-2, it may reduce general inflammation, which may be linked with Alzheimer's disease in an as yet unidentified manner.
3. By reducing the risk of embolism formation in people with low risk atrial fibrillation (see page 100), it may reduce the risk of some types of vascular dementia.

## What the research says

In 1996, a review[33] was made of seventeen studies from nine countries. These studies examined whether the use of anti-inflammatory drugs was a protective factor for Alzheimer's disease. Such use had been associated with a reduced prevalence of Alzheimer's. This would be entirely in keeping with the premise that Alzheimer's disease is a form of inflammation of the brain, or that it is associated in some way with an inflammatory process.

The review found that although many of the trials were small, there was sufficient evidence to suggest that anti-inflammatory drugs (NSAIDs, of which aspirin is one) might have a protective effect against Alzheimer's disease.

### The Cache County Study[34]

Between 1995 and 1996, patients aged 65 years and above, residents of Cache County, were assessed for evidence of dementia, and for their use of NSAIDs, including aspirin, as well as for various other drugs. Three years later, the researchers obtained further medical histories and found:

- 104 of 3,227 patients who were still living had developed Alzheimer's disease.
- The incidence of Alzheimer's disease was marginally reduced in those using NSAIDs at any time.
- Increased duration of use was associated with a greater reduction.
- Similar patterns were noted for aspirin usage.

The study was published in 2002 and concluded that long-term use of NSAIDs and aspirin may reduce the incidence of Alzheimer's disease, provided that the use has started well before the onset of dementia.

### Women's Health Study Cognitive Cohort

This was a large study with a negative finding, which was published in 2007.[35] Over a ten-year period, 6,377 women were studied to investigate the effect of aspirin on their cognitive function. The patients were randomized – half to receive low dose aspirin (100mg) and half placebo. Cognitive functioning was not found to be significantly different in the two groups. The researchers concluded that no apparent benefit was seen in taking aspirin.

## The US Veterans Study

This study, published in 2008[36], looked at whether NSAIDs taken for 5 years or more could reduce the incidence of Alzheimer's disease.

* 49,349 cases with Alzheimer's disease were recruited using the US Veterans Affairs Health Care system.
* 196,850 controls were also identified.
* Researchers looked at the usage of long-term NSAIDs in both groups.
* NSAID usage reduced the risk of Alzheimer's disease.
* Ibuprofen seemed to be the most effective drug.

The researchers concluded that long-term use of anti-inflammatory drugs (NSAIDs) *was* protective against Alzheimer's disease, with ibuprofen seeming to be particularly effective.

## Six Pooled Cohort Studies

Also published in 2008 was this paper from the Johns Hopkins Bloomberg School of Public Health and researchers from elsewhere around the US.[37] They pooled data from six prospective studies to examine the risk of Alzheimer's disease in users of various kinds of anti-inflammatory drugs.

Previous researchers had suggested that a sub-group of NSAIDs, known as the SALAs (e.g. diclofenac and ibuprofen), might be more effective than other types of NSAID. The SALAs act by selectively lowering levels of the peptide beta-amyloid, which has been found in the brains of Alzheimer's patients.

- Researchers examined the data from 13,499 people who had no history of Alzheimer's disease at entry to the studies.
- 820 people developed Alzheimer's disease during the course of the studies.
- NSAIDs reduced the risk of developing the disease by 23 per cent.
- There was no difference between NSAIDs. The SALAs were no more effective than the others, including aspirin.
- Aspirin gave the same level of reduction of 23 per cent.

Conclusion: aspirin was just as effective as other NSAIDs at reducing the risk of developing Alzheimer's disease, reducing the risk by 23 per cent.

### CHAPTER SUMMARY

Research suggests that Alzheimer's disease may be an inflammatory condition, so it makes sense that aspirin, an anti-inflammatory drug, would be effective in treating it. However, there is conflicting evidence from the various trials. Some are very positive and suggest that aspirin and other NSAIDs do have a protective effect, whereas others suggest no effect.

While the negative results temper a definitive conclusion, there is certainly enough positive evidence for a discussion about whether aspirin would be a sensible drug for the individual who is concerned about their risk of developing Alzheimer's disease, providing there is no contraindication. After all:

- In the studies reviewed in this chapter, four out of five suggested that aspirin use could reduce the risk of developing Alzheimer's disease.

# ASPIRIN AND DEMENTIA

- One study suggested it could reduce the risk by as much as **23 per cent**.

However, do note: for any benefit, it seems that aspirin has to be taken long term, probably for at least 5 years, and *before* the onset of dementia.

Aspirin also has a role to play in preventing vascular dementia, the second most common form of dementia after Alzheimer's disease. Vascular dementia is primarily caused by strokes in the brain. As stroke prevention will limit the risks of vascular dementia, aspirin – already shown to be effective at preventing strokes – may also prevent vascular dementia, primarily in those people who are at increased risk of having a stroke or a heart attack, as defined in previous chapters.

# CANCER: A SHORT OVERVIEW

## 10

Cancer is not a single disease, but the name for a group of diseases. There are over 200 types that are recognized. Each type is classified according to the type of cell from which it arose.

Essentially, a cancer occurs when cells do not die, but grow and reproduce out of control and out of phase from the rest of the body.

## Cancer statistics

- One person in three will develop cancer at some stage in their life.
- Four cancers – breast, bowel, lung and prostate – account for 54 per cent of new cancers.
- 64 per cent of new cancers occur in people of 65 years and older.
- Less that 1 per cent of cancers develop in children aged 0–14 years.
- Breast cancer is the commonest cancer in the UK, despite being rare in men.
- Globally, the most common causes of cancer death are cancer of the lung, cancer of the stomach and cancer of the liver.

- Cancer of unknown primary – an advanced cancer at diagnosis, but when the site of the original tumour and its type are not known – accounts for 4 per cent of new cancers.
- Globally, there are an estimated 12.7 million new cases of cancer diagnosed each year.
- Globally, there are 7.6 million cancer deaths a year.

## Normal growth and repair

The average adult human body is made up of about 25–100 trillion* cells. The cells are the basic building blocks of the body. Groups of cells are arranged into different types of tissue, and various tissues make up the individual organs of the body.

Throughout the whole of life, there is an amazing continuous programme of growth and repair of organs and tissues going on. This involves the cells of each tissue living, performing their necessary functions for a programmed length of time, and then dying. As they get old or if they get damaged, they die and are replaced by new ones being developed to take their place.

This happens in a superbly coordinated manner. Most cells are programmed to divide in a well ordered and controlled manner, so that new cells take the place of ones that die and are removed.

## Tumour formation

If the normal growth and repair cycle goes wrong, then some cells may not die off, but continue to live and keep on dividing to produce an abnormal mass of cells. This can form into a lump called a tumour. This can happen in any part of the body.

* A trillion is 1 million million.

A tumour may cause problems by growing large and pressing on neighbouring tissues or organs. As a result, it may interfere with the function of the nervous, digestive, circulatory or respiratory systems. Some tumours may even pump out hormones which have an unwanted and destabilizing effect on the body.

There are two types of tumour:

- Benign – these stay in one place, do not pump out any hormones and only produce a problem by pressing on neighbouring structures.
- Malignant – these are made of cells that have the ability to move around the body via the blood and the lymphatic systems. **Malignant tumours are referred to as cancers.**

---

### THE LYMPHATIC SYSTEM

The lymphatic system is a system of very fine tubes called lymphatic vessels that link up to various lymph nodes throughout the body. Its purpose is to carry lymph or lymphatic fluid containing white blood cells to all of the tissues, rather like the way that the circulation carries blood. The tonsils, adenoids, thymus gland and spleen are all glands of the lymphatic system and together they form the bulk of your immune system.

---

## The spread of a cancer

Malignant tumours are dangerous because they can spread. The originating tumour is referred to as a primary tumour.

- If cancerous cells spread to another part of the body, the process is called metastasis.
- A metastasis is also the name given to a localization of cells that have spread from a primary tumour. Thus, a metastasis is a secondary tumour and the primary tumour is said to have metastasized.
- If there are multiple secondary tumours, then the condition is referred to as metastatic cancer, meaning that there is a primary tumour and multiple secondary tumours.

Two processes are involved:

- *Invasion* – when cancerous cells break loose from a primary tumour and grow into neighbouring tissues (local invasion), then spread to another part of the body via the bloodstream or the lymphatic system. They may then start to grow by repeated cell divisions. This further destroys the normal tissues that it invades.
- *Angiogenesis* – the cancerous cells stimulate growth of blood vessels, so that they effectively develop their own blood supply, which will supply them with the nutrients that they need to grow.

Metastasis can occur to different tissues. Different cancers have different tendencies to spread. For example, cancers of the lung, breast, thyroid, prostate and kidney can all spread to bones. Gastrointestinal cancers and pancreatic cancers may spread to the liver. Cancers of the colon, kidney and malignant melanomas (skin cancer) may spread to the brain.

## The symptoms of cancer

These are highly variable. There may be symptoms:

- Associated with the primary tumour if it is altering the structure of the local tissues or pressing on an organ and

altering its function. For example, a cancerous tumour of the colon may cause a sudden alteration of the person's bowel habit. A cancer of the lung may produce a persistent cough. A cancer of the uterus may cause unexpected vaginal bleeding.
* Associated with metastasis. For example, secondary deposits in bones may result in extreme bone pain. Secondaries in the brain may produce psychological and cognitive changes.
* Associated with inflammatory changes that seem to be triggered off. It is common to find that certain blood tests register that inflammation is present somewhere.
* Associated with inappropriate secretion of hormones, so that a hormonal disease may be the first sign of an underlying malignancy.
* Associated with metabolic changes as the result of the malignancy process. This may result in the individual's general energy levels dropping, they may feel nauseated, generally unwell, feverish and lose weight.

## The causes of cancer

There are lots of things that seem to have the potential to cause normal cells to become cancerous. Anything that can cause a change in the DNA of the cell may turn it into a cancerous cell. A cancerous cell does not die, but continues to divide and forms new cells that function autonomously and which do not serve the body any useful purpose.

### Carcinogens

These are chemicals or agents that seem to have a direct poisonous effect on cells, resulting in damage to the DNA.

That said, not all of them cause DNA damage and instead cause cancerous change by inducing mutations in ways that are not fully understood. One way that is known is by simply causing an increase in cell divisions. When that happens, there is an increased likelihood of producing a mutation.

Some known carcinogens are:

- Tobacco products and tobacco smoke
- Radiation
- Solar radiation
- Arsenic
- Beryllium
- Asbestos
- Cadmium
- Various organic dyes and chemicals

## Genes

There are four types of genes that play a major role in cell division. This seems to be one of the crucial parts in the process.

If these genes are impeded, then they will not take part in the normal processes of growth and repair, and cancer may be the result.

- Oncogenes – these instruct cells on when they should divide. If this function is impeded by mutation then there will be uncontrolled and uncoordinated cell divisions, out of phase with the rest of the body.
- Tumour suppressor genes – sometimes called anti-oncogenes, these instruct cells when they should *not* divide. When this function is impeded by mutation, cells will continue to divide and tumour formation is more likely.
- Suicide genes – these instruct cells when they should die. They are activated when a cell is showing DNA damage and the body needs to remove it. This process of cell death is called *apoptosis*. If this function is suppressed, the cell will not kill itself and will go on living.

- DNA repair genes – these instruct a cell to initiate repair of damaged DNA. If these genes do not work, a cell will not be able to correct the mutation that it is and will continue to reproduce the mutation through further cell divisions.

## Familial tendency

This is also a problem that is brought about through the genetic material that one has inherited. Some genes may be switched on and others switched off, thereby making the individual more susceptible to the development of cancer.

Bowel cancer is such a condition that may seem to run in families. There are certain genes that may be tested for. For example:

- Familial adenomatous polyposis – the APC gene – a rare condition that causes 1 per cent of bowel cancers.
- Lynch syndrome or hereditary non-polyposis colon cancer – an inherited disorder of three DNA repair genes. It causes 2–5 per cent of bowel cancers. It is also associated with an increased risk of developing small bowel, liver, gall bladder, ovarian, uterine and brain cancers.

## Non-specific inflammation

The role of inflammation in cancer is gaining more and more attention. As we know from previous chapters in this book, prostaglandins are involved in inflammation – and there is accumulating evidence that they are involved in polyp (tumour) formation in the colon. We shall look at this in the next chapter.

## Slow viruses

There are several viruses which have been associated with the development of some cancers.

Viruses consist of strands of DNA or RNA*, usually surrounded by a protein coat. They do not live independently, but take over the DNA of cells that they invade, making them reproduce copies of the virus. The body gradually overcomes this process, but some of the virus DNA or RNA may become included in host cells' nucleic acid, causing a tendency to mutation later on.

Some of the viruses that have cancer associations are:

- HPV – human papilloma virus, which is linked with cancer of the cervix
- Epstein-Barr virus, associated with some childhood cancers, Burkitt's lymphoma, Hodgkin's disease, post-transplantation lymphoma and naso-pharyngeal cancer
- Hepatitis B and hepatitis C, and liver cancer

## Classification of cancer

It is important to classify cancer in order to choose the most appropriate type of treatment. The following are the main categories of cancer.

- Carcinomas – these are malignancies arising from epithelial cells, or the type of cells that line or cover internal organs and form the skin.
- Sarcomas – these are malignancies arising from connective tissue cells, such as from bone, cartilage, muscle, fat or fibrous tissue.
- Lymphomas and myelomas – these are malignancies arising from the lymphatic tissue of the immune system.

* DNA and RNA are nucleic acids. DNA (Desoxyribose Nucleic Acid) is the double-stranded nucleic acid that contains the genetic information in each cell of every living organsism, which determines the development and the function of the cell. RNA is the single-stranded nucleic acid that transports messages within the cell.

- Leukaemias – these are malignancies of the blood and the blood-forming tissues of the body. There may not be tumour formation, but there is abnormal production of various types of blood cell. Organs like the spleen and liver may be affected and lymph glands around the body may be affected.
- Central nervous system – these are malignancies arising from cells in the brain or spinal cord.

## The stages of cancer

It is vitally important to stage a cancer in order to determine how a treatment can be tailored to suit the individual's need. The earlier a cancer is diagnosed, the better. Cancer that has metastasized (spread to another part of the body) is harder to treat.

A whole host of special investigations may be needed, including blood tests, X-rays, ultrasound scans, CT scans, and MRI scans. Various endoscopic investigations may be used, in which a fibre-optic scope is introduced into the body to provide visual examination and also to facilitate the taking of biopsies.

Microscopic examination of cells removed in a process called biopsying may give the definitive diagnosis.

### The systems used to stage cancer

There are two main systems used to stage a cancer.

*The TNM system*

This stands for Tumour, Nodes and Metastasis. Each of these is given a grading so that a doctor can describe the size of the primary tumour, whether there are nodes that the cancer has spread to, and whether the cancer has spread to other parts of the body. This system is used with breast, lung and colorectal cancer.

Colorectal cancer is *also* graded by the Duke's system, whereby the letters A, B, C and D give an indication of how far the cancer has spread. Grade A means that it is only affecting the innermost layer of the bowel. Grades B and C refer to progressively further spread, which is still treatable by operation. Grade D refers to cancer that has already spread to distant parts of the body like the liver and the lungs.

*Number systems*

These are used with certain types of cancer. Usually there are four gradations used, from 1 to 4, with stage 4 cancer being the most serious. Cancer of the uterus is graded in this way, as are liver cancer and lymphomas.

## The treatment of cancer

This very much depends upon the type of cancer and its stage, and upon the age, general health and strength of the individual. There may well be a principal treatment which is then backed up with one or two other types of treatment. Treatment may be aimed at curing the cancer or it may be palliative (relieving pain without tackling the cause of the condition).

Treatments may involve:

- Surgery – to remove a primary tumour or to improve the function of a part of the body. Generally, this is more likely to be an option if metastasis has not taken place.
- Radiotherapy – this is the irradiation of the tumour with focused high-energy radiation, with the intention of killing cancerous cells. It may be combined with chemotherapy for some types of cancer, such as the breast in some cases.
- Chemotherapy – the use of powerful drugs that interfere with the metabolism of the cancer cells, causing them to die or to commit suicide.

- Other treatments – hormone therapy may help in certain hormonally dependent cancers. Immunotherapy by stimulating the immune system may help. Gene therapy may have great promise in the future.

## General measures to prevent cancer

It is recognized that one third of cancers are preventable by lifestyle change.

### Tobacco

This is the largest preventable cause of cancer throughout the world.

- It causes 80–90 per cent of all lung cancer deaths.
- It causes 30 per cent of all cancer deaths in developing countries.
- The WHO (World Health Organization) is committed to reducing cancer deaths and the WHO Framework Convention on Tobacco Control was adopted in May 2003. It has been signed by 168 countries and is legally binding in 172 countries. It lays down restrictions on tobacco usage. It is perhaps one of the most important public health measures of all time.

### Diet

A good wholesome diet is essential for good health.

- Obesity is associated with cancers of the oesophagus, colorectum, breast, endometrium and kidney.
- Diets rich in fruit and vegetables may be protective against many cancers.
- Diets rich in red meat may be associated with colorectal cancer.

## Exercise

This is known to be good for general health and well-being.

- It is good for cardio-respiratory function and fitness, which may have a protective effect in its own right.
- Regular exercise is likely to help individuals to avoid obesity.

## Infections

It is known that certain infectious organisms can predispose towards cancers. Measures to avoid such infections should be taken.

- Viral Hepatitis B and Hepatitis C are associated with cancer of the liver.
- Human papilloma virus is associated with cancer of the cervix.
- Helicobacter pylori is associated with an increased risk of stomach cancer. This bug also causes stomach ulceration and a lot of stomach complaints. It can be detected by blood testing or a breath test.
- In some countries, schistosomiasis is associated with bladder cancer. It is also called bilharziosis or snail fever and is a parasitic worm infestation common in the tropics. It needs to be considered in anyone returning from the tropics.

## Solar radiation

It is well documented that excessive exposure to solar radiation can induce all types of skin cancer. It is sensible to use sunscreens when exposed to the sun.

## Occupational risks

Certain occupations are associated with increased risk of certain cancers.

- In 1981, Doll and Peto[38] reported to the US Congress that about 4 per cent of cancers were attributable to occupation.
- Asbestos has been the biggest industrial carcinogen.
- It is extremely hard to diagnose and prove an occupational cause.

## Aspirin and cancer prevention

Various lines of research suggest that aspirin may have a part to play in preventing some cancers.

### Animal studies

The COX-2 enzyme (introduced on page 49) has been looked at as a potential target for cancer prevention[39], with the following results:

- Raised levels of the COX-2 enzyme have been found in pre-malignant and malignant tissues.
- Experimental animals which have been bred to be COX-2 deficient have been shown to have reduced tumour formation and growth.
- Experimental animals that have been treated with selective COX-2 inhibitors have shown reduced tumour formation and growth.

In the mid-1970s, researchers found that prostaglandin $E_2$ levels were raised in malignant tumours from the rectum and colon. Prostaglandin $E_2$ has been identified as one of the main prostaglandins associated with inflammation.

This led to a spate of experiments in which NSAIDs (Non-Steroidal Anti-Inflammatory Drugs, such as aspirin and ibuprofen) were shown to reduce or inhibit tumours that had been chemically induced in rats and mice.

These animal experiments proved conclusively that aspirin and other NSAIDs could inhibit experimentally induced cancers in rats and mice.

## Cell research

In 1998, researchers at several centres[40] investigated both COX-1 and COX-2 effects and postulated that aspirin works by two methods in reducing the risk of cancer:

- COX-2 inhibition – this prevents cancer cells from initiating new blood vessel growth (angiogenesis – see page 129). This means the tumour is not able to set up its own blood supply and 'feed' itself.
- COX-1 inhibition – this could have an effect on the epithelial lining cells of blood vessels, inhibiting growth of blood vessels into the tumour, meaning once again that the tumour will lack the nutrients it needs in order to grow, as it will not have a ready supply of blood.

## Observational studies in humans

Several studies of people in the general population who regularly use aspirin have shown a lower incidence of adenomatous polyps (defined in the box below) in the bowel and a lower incidence of cancer of the colon and of death from cancer of the colon, compared with non-users of aspirin.

In fact, long-term use of NSAIDs is associated with a 30–50 per cent reduction in the incidence of polyps, cancer of the colon and death in all but one study that was reviewed.[41] These results strongly support the hypothesis that aspirin and NSAIDs could reduce the occurrence or the onward progression of cancer of the colon in the general population.

Significantly, the observational studies suggested that aspirin needs to be taken for at least 5 years before an effect is seen in a reduction of the risk of cancer.

> ### ADENOMAS AND ADENOMATOUS TUMOURS
>
> - An adenoma is a tumour arising from glandular tissue. They can occur in all manner of organs.
> - An adenomatous polyp is another name for an adenoma. It is benign.
> - An adenocarcinoma is a *malignant* tumour arising from glandular tissue in an organ. Wherever 'carcinoma' makes the second part of a word, it means that it is a cancer and it is malignant.

## Aspirin and long-term risk of death due to cancer

At the end of 2010 and the beginning of 2011, two major papers were published in *The Lancet*.

The first was a follow-up of five randomized trials in which aspirin was used.[42] It showed that the long-term use of daily low dose aspirin of 75–300mg reduced the risk of death from cancer of the colon by a third. We shall look at this in more detail in the chapter on Colorectal cancer.

The second was an analysis of eight studies involving 25,570 patients, which had originally been conducted to determine the protective effect of low-dose aspirin on cardio-vascular disease.[43] Several of these trials we have previously considered in the chapters on the heart and circulation.

## The trials

The trials analysed in the second study were:

* British Doctors Aspirin Trial (BDAT)
* UK Transient Ischaemic Attack Trial (UK-TIA)
* Early Treatment Diabetic Retinopathy Study (ETDRS)
* Swedish Angina Pectoris Aspirin Trial (SAPAT)
* Thrombosis Prevention Trial (TPT)
* Japanese Primary Prevention of Atherosclerosis with Aspirin for Diabetes (JPAD)
* Prevention of Progression of Arterial Disease and Diabetes (POPADAD)
* Aspirin for Asymptomatic Atherosclerosis (AAA)

Three of the trials had continued to obtain data for deaths from cancer after completion of the trials, by the national death certification and the cancer registration systems. These were: Thrombosis Prevention Trial (TPT); British Doctors Aspirin Trial (BDAT) and UK Transient Ischaemic Attack Trial (UK-TIA).

* The research trials had been carried on from 4 to 8 years.
* Patients were followed up for up to 20 years after.
* During the trials, overall cancer death rate fell by 21 per cent in the aspirin users.

## Analysing the results

* The benefit for some cancers did not appear until the user had been taking the aspirin for 5 years.
* After 5 years of taking aspirin, the death rate for all cancers fell by 34 per cent.
* After 5 years of taking aspirin, the death rate for gastrointestinal cancers fell by 54 per cent.
* The risk for stomach and colorectal cancers fell after 10 years.

- Aspirin reduced deaths due to primary brain tumours during the first 10 years of follow-up.
- The risk for prostate cancers fell after 15 years.
- There was no difference with dose, sex, smoking.
- Benefit increased with age – the longer it had been taken, the better, up to 20–25 years of use.

Death rates dropped after 20 years of aspirin use:

- The overall risk of cancer death was reduced by 20 per cent over a 20-year period.
- By 10 per cent for prostate cancer.
- By 30 per cent for lung cancer (but only for the adenocarcinoma type, which is more common in non-smokers).
- By 40 per cent for colorectal cancer.
- By 60 per cent for oesophageal cancer (of adenocarcinoma type).

## More research needed

- The effect on stomach, pancreatic and brain cancers was hard to determine, since insufficient numbers were seen to do a clear statistical analysis.
- There was no significant effect on haematological cancers (cancers of the blood).
- There were too few women in the trials to determine the effects of aspirin on breast cancer or gynaecological cancers.

## The type of cancerous change seems critical

Cancer change can occur in any type of cell that makes up a tissue.

- Squamous cell carcinoma is a cancer arising from squamous epithelial cells. These are flat, pavement-like cells that

line tubes or hollow organs like the kidneys, lungs or the bladder, or the surface of the skin, the mouth, the oesophagus and the lips.
- Adenocarcinomas are cancers that arise from adenomatous or glandular cells that line various tubes or organs.

Some cancers can be either squamous cell carcinomas or adenocarcinomas. Oesophageal cancer and lung cancer can be either type.

In the study, it seemed that aspirin *only* had an effect in reducing deaths from adenocarcinomas, rather than other types of cancer, such as squamous cell carcinoma. This is especially noticeable in cancer of the lung and oesophagus, but also of relevance in other cancers where adenocarcinoma predominates over other cancerous change, such as the stomach, small bowel, colon, rectum, pancreas, breast, ovary and prostate.

### CHAPTER SUMMARY

- Long-term aspirin use is associated with an overall reduction in the risk of several cancers, including cancers of the colon, rectum, stomach, bowel, lung, oesophagus, prostate and brain. The benefit was consistent across *all* of the studies.
- The effect takes 5 years to become apparent.
- There seems to be a greater effect in reducing the risk of certain cancers, in particular gastrointestinal cancer, for which death rates were reduced by **54 per cent**.
- **The overall cancer death rate was reduced by 34 per cent after 5 years of aspirin use.**
- There is no difference in aspirin dose – 75mg seems sufficient to produce the effect.
- The longer the usage, the greater the reduction in risk: 20–25

years of usage gives the best protection. After that, there may be more risk of haemorrhages.
- The peak time to start to reap the benefit seems to be when patients are in their late forties and fifties.

# 11
# COLORECTAL CANCER

The term colorectal cancer means cancer affecting the colon, the large bowel and the rectum, the last few inches of the large bowel.

## The colon – more than just a tube

The word 'colon' comes from the Greek *kolon*. The term was introduced by Aristotle, the Greek philosopher and anatomist, in the fourth century BC.

It is a large muscular tube that connects the small intestine to the rectum. It is a surprising five feet in length, and is curled up inside the abdomen in a series of twists and turns, prior to ending in the rectum.

Its functions are:

- To absorb water, minerals and salts from the partially digested food that it receives from the small intestine. Two pints of liquid matter enter it each day and about one third of a pint will enter the rectum. The rest is re-absorbed by the colon.
- To transport this matter down along its length to the rectum by muscular contractions, which take place several times a day.

- To help with the ongoing degradation and digestion of the food, by virtue of the huge number of micro-organisms, the bowel microflora, which it contains.

## The rectum – not just a straight tube

In fact, the rectum is not straight at all, which is at variance with its name, which is from the Latin *rectus*, meaning 'straight'. It was given this name by the physician and anatomist Claudius Galen in the first century, because in dissections of animals he had found it to be straight.

It is a muscular tube about six inches long. It joins the sigmoid colon (the part of the colon that forms a repository for faecal matter) just above the pelvis, and it travels down through the pelvis to the anal canal. It has three curves.

Its function is to store faeces and gas. It is able to expand so it can hold a considerable amount of matter until the individual chooses to expel it.

## Colorectal cancer

Cancer can affect any part of the body, but some parts with greater frequency than others. Cancer of the small intestine is rare, but colorectal cancer is relatively common.

According to Cancer Research (UK):

- Colorectal cancer is more common in developed countries than in underdeveloped countries.
- Globally, there are about 1 million new cases each year.
- Globally, there are about 600,000 deaths from colorectal cancer each year.
- 106 new cases of colorectal cancer are diagnosed in the UK every day.
- Colorectal cancer is the third most common cancer in the UK after breast and lung cancer.

**COLORECTAL CANCER**

- In 2007, there were 38,608 new cases of colorectal cancer registered in the UK. Two thirds (24,274) were in the colon and one third (14,334) were in the rectum.
- Cancer of the distal colon and rectum are far commoner than of the proximal colon.*
- Most colorectal cancers develop from adenomatous polyps (defined on page 140).
- Colorectal cancer is strongly age-linked: 84 per cent of cases arise after the age of 65 years.
- The lifetime risk of developing colorectal cancer is 1 in 16 for men and 1 in 20 for women.

# Risk factors for colorectal cancer

- Increasing age
- Positive family history
- Genetic predisposition
  1. Familial adenomatous polyposis – the APC gene – a rare condition that causes 1 per cent of bowel cancers.
  2. Lynch syndrome or hereditary non-polyposis colon cancer
- Inflammatory bowel disease – ulcerative colitis or Crohn's disease
- Obesity
- Lifestyle – smoking, sedentary, poor diet, excess alcohol

# Protective factors

- HRT for women
- Good diet with lots of fruit and vegetables
- Good diet with restricted red meat
- **Long-term use of aspirin or NSAIDs**

---

* Proximal means nearest the start, so proximal colon means nearest the start of the colon, i.e. nearest the small intestine. Distal means furthest from the start, so distal colon means the descending colon and rectum.

## Aspirin and colorectal cancer

Several studies have looked at whether aspirin can help in tackling colorectal cancer. What is particularly encouraging about its interaction with this particular cancer is that the signs are strong that it could help with both primary and secondary prevention. So what has the research shown so far?

## Primary prevention

Laboratory and epidemiological research had been suggestive that aspirin and other NSAIDs had an anti-tumour effect in the large bowel. A trial published in the *New England Journal of Medicine* in 2003 by a group of researchers set out to see if this could actually be the case.[44]

They performed a randomized double-blind trial of aspirin as a chemical preventive of adenomatous polyp formation. An adenomatous polyp is benign, not malignant. The importance of being able to prevent them, of course, is the fact that most colorectal cancers develop from an adenomatous polyp.

An adenomatous polyp can become an adenocarcinoma (malignant tumour) at any time. We don't know when that occurs. In some people, it never happens. In others, it may happen at once. That is why a polyp needs to be removed, in case it is cancerous. If it is, then the person has cancer and needs treatment. If not, then they just need follow-up treatment to make sure they don't develop further polyps.

- 1,121 patients were enrolled on the trial, all of whom had previously been found to have a bowel polyp.
- They were randomized to receive either:
  o Placebo
  o Low dose of aspirin – 81mg
  o Standard aspirin – 325mg
- Follow-up colonoscopy was performed after 3 years.

Researchers found that the incidence of one or more adenomas was:

- 47 per cent in the placebo group
- 38 per cent in the low dose aspirin group
- 45 per cent in the standard aspirin group

They concluded that low dose aspirin has a moderate effect in preventing adenomatous polyps in the colon.

## Secondary prevention

Another trial was performed to see whether aspirin could prevent the formation of adenomatous polyps in patients who had previously been treated for colorectal cancer.[45] This was a most important question to look at. Researchers conducted a randomized double-blind trial on the effect of aspirin on the incidence of colonic polyps.

- 635 patients were enrolled on the trial, all of whom had previously been diagnosed with and treated for colorectal cancer.
- They were randomized to either receive 325mg aspirin daily or a placebo.
- The trial was ended before its due date because statistically significant results were found at an interim analysis.
- They found that the incidence of one or more polyps was:
  o 17 per cent in the aspirin group
  o 27 per cent in the placebo group
- They also discovered that the time taken to develop an adenomatous polyp was much longer in the aspirin group.

Conclusion: daily use of aspirin is associated with a significant reduction in the incidence of adenomatous polyps in patients who have a history of colonic cancer.

## Long-term studies

These were amazingly important findings, yet they were trials that had only been carried out over a short period of a few years. What was needed was an idea of what would happen over a much longer period of time.

An analysis of the results obtained from two large trials on the use of aspirin in the prevention of vascular events, which had been followed up for several more years, gave some idea. The follow-up results from the British Doctors Aspirin Trial (BDAT) and the UK Transient Ischaemic Attack Trial (UK-TIA) showed that daily high dose aspirin (500mg or more) for more than 5 years was associated with a reduction in the incidence of colorectal cancer after a latent period of about 10 years.[46] In other words, it seemed to take 10 years before an effect became apparent.

## The dosage question

What hadn't yet been proved conclusively was what level of dosage was required to exact a beneficial response in a patient. This is a particularly important concern in the case of aspirin because it was known that the risk of having a significant bleed (a possible side effect of the drug) is related to the dose. The greater the dose, the more likely a haemorrhage is.

There was therefore a need to know what the minimum dose would be that would have a beneficial effect. In addition, it was desirable to know whether the beneficial effect was dose-related. Was the effect better the higher the dose?

## The big analysis

In October 2010, a major piece of research was published in *The Lancet* by Professor Peter Rothwell and colleagues. It was called: 'Long-term effect of aspirin on colorectal cancer incidence and mortality: 20-year follow-up of five randomized trials.'[47]

They followed up four large randomized trials of aspirin versus controls in the primary and secondary prevention of vascular events, and one trial of different doses of aspirin. Their purpose was to see whether or not aspirin could reduce the incidence of colorectal cancer during the trials and over a 20-year period of follow-up.

They analysed the pooled patient data from all five trials* to form their conclusions.

They found:

- 391 (2.8 per cent) of 14,033 patients developed colorectal cancer during follow-up over the 20 years.
- Allocation to the aspirin group reduced the 20-year risk of colon cancer – but not rectal cancer.
- Where information about the position of the cancer was available, aspirin reduced the risk of proximal colon cancer – but not distal colon cancer.
- With aspirin usage of 5 years or more, aspirin reduced the risk of proximal colon cancer by 70 per cent and also reduced the risk of rectal cancer.
- No benefit was seen at doses greater than 75mg daily.
- There was a risk of fatal colorectal cancer when the aspirin dosage was only 30mg (as found on the Dutch TIA trial).

Conclusion: aspirin has a major beneficial effect in reducing the risk of colorectal cancer when taken as a daily 75mg dose for at least 5 years.

* Primary prevention: Thrombosis Prevention Trial (TPT), British Doctors Aspirin Trial (BDAT); secondary prevention: UK Transient Ischaemic Attack Trial (UK-TIA), Swedish Aspirin Low Dose Trial; different dose trial: Dutch TIA Aspirin Trial.

## CHAPTER SUMMARY

The 2010 aspirin study is an incredibly important piece of scientific evidence. It proves that long-term low dose aspirin use can benefit patients by reducing the risk of colorectal cancer – for certain types by as much as **70 per cent**.

It also gives a way of preventing proximal colorectal cancer, which is difficult to diagnose because it is not easy to screen for or view by sigmoidoscopy or colonoscopy*, whereas distal cancers are. This is significant because a cancer that is hard to diagnose may not be caught in time and later treatment may prove ineffective. To prevent the cancer from developing in the first place is, of course, the preferred scenario, and aspirin potentially gives us that option.

Aspirin use has also been shown to have an effect on reducing the incidence of adenomatous polyps, which can lead to colorectal cancer. There was a moderate primary prevention success rate, and a significant secondary prevention effect for patients who already had a history of polyps.

There is therefore very good reason in my opinion why anyone at risk – provided as usual that there are no contraindications – should consider with their doctor taking regular daily low dose aspirin.

There is also a case for anyone over the age of fifty – who has no contraindications – considering with their doctor the use of regular daily low dose aspirin as a means of reducing their risk of colorectal cancer.

---

* Sigmoidoscopy and colonoscopy are both endoscopic procedures, whereby a fibre-optic microscope is inserted into the body for interior visual examination.

# CANCER OF THE LUNG 12

Lung cancer is one of the commonest and most dangerous cancers.

Shockingly, three quarters of all lung cancer patients die within 12 months of their diagnosis.

Cancer that begins in the lungs is called primary lung cancer, as opposed to secondary cancer, which is cancer that has spread from another organ.

## Types of lung cancer

There are two types of primary lung cancer, which are classified according to the type of cell that it starts in:

1. Non-small cell carcinoma – 80 per cent of lung cancers, of which there are three types: squamous cell carcinoma, adenocarcinoma and large cell carcinoma.
2. Small cell carcinoma – 20 per cent of lung cancers. It is also known as oat cell carcinoma. This tends to be more aggressive and spreads faster.

## Some facts about lung cancer

- It is the second most common cancer in the UK.
- It is the most common cause of cancer-related deaths in both men and women.
- In 2007, there were 29,600 lung cancer deaths in England and Wales.
- Tobacco-smoking is the single biggest cause of lung cancer, in about 90–95 per cent of cases.
- People who smoke twenty or more cigarettes a day are twenty times more likely to develop lung cancer than non-smokers.
- Only 25 per cent of people diagnosed with lung cancer will survive longer than a year.

## Aspirin and lung cancer

Although information had been coming out about aspirin's potential benefit in preventing other cancers, there was little information until the early noughties about any use with lung cancer.

### New York Women's Health Study

In 2002, a study was published in the *British Journal of Cancer* that looked hopeful.[48] The association between aspirin usage and lung cancer risk was examined in a nested* case control study in the New York Women's Health Study.

- 81 cases of lung cancer developed in the cohort.
- They each matched with ten controls from the cohort, for age, menopausal status, dates of enrolment and follow-up.

* A nested study means that a group of patients with a specified disease are selected from a well-defined cohort (sample) of people. They are then compared with a group of people without the disease, who had also been included within the cohort.

They found a strong inverse relationship between those who used aspirin three times a week for six months or more, compared to non-aspirin users. This means that those who used aspirin had a much lower risk of developing lung cancer.

## BMC Cancer Study

Another study was published in *BMC Cancer* in 2003.[49] These researchers conducted a hospital-based case-control study to evaluate whether regular usage of aspirin could be protective against the development of lung cancer.

- 868 patients had developed lung cancer.
- They were matched with 935 patients who had been treated for non-cancer conditions.
- They all completed comprehensive questionnaires covering family, occupational and environmental history, the use of tobacco, alcohol, and dietary pattern. In addition, they answered questions about aspirin usage, how much was taken, how often, and duration of use.
- Average age was 62 years.
- 60 per cent were men and 40 per cent women.

The researchers found that regular aspirin users (defined as those who used aspirin at least once a week for at least one year) had a significantly lower rate of lung cancer, for both small cell and non-small cell carcinomas.

## The large study

The biggest study of the effect of aspirin on lung cancer to date was the meta-analysis published in *The Lancet* in January 2011, entitled 'Effect of daily aspirin on long-term risk of death due to cancer: analysis of individual patient data from randomized trials'. It found that there *was* a reduction in the risk of death from lung cancer – but it does take 5 years to become apparent.

For adenocarcinoma, the reduction in death risk was 30 per cent. There was no reduction noticed for small cell or squamous cell carcinomas.

### CHAPTER SUMMARY

- There certainly is evidence that aspirin reduces the risk of primary lung cancer, but mainly adenocarcinoma, which is more common in non-smokers. The most recent research suggests a reduction in the death rate of 30 per cent for adenocarcinomas.
- It would be worth discussing this research with your doctor if there is a family history of lung cancer.
- Anyone who smokes is strongly advised to quit the habit as soon as possible, for that is the single best thing that can be done to reduce risk.

# BREAST CANCER 13

The possibility of developing breast cancer is a great anxiety to most women.

## Some basic statistics

According to Cancer Research UK:

- Breast cancer is the most common cancer in the UK.
- The lifetime risk of developing breast cancer for women in the UK is 1 in 8.
- Female breast cancer incidence rates in Great Britain have increased by more than 50 per cent in the past 25 years.
- Currently about 130 women in the UK are diagnosed with breast cancer every day.
- 80 per cent of breast cancers occur in women over the age of 50 years.
- About 340 men develop breast cancer in any year.
- Globally, there are about 11.38 million cases of breast cancer diagnosed each year.
- Breast cancer survival rates have been improving over the last 40 years.
- Women diagnosed today are twice as likely to survive for at least 10 years than 40 years ago.

## Aspirin and breast cancer

There have been many studies over the years that suggest a place for aspirin in the prevention of breast cancer.

### Risk reduction?

In 2008, researchers from Guy's and St Thomas' Hospital Trust published a paper in the *International Journal of Clinical Practice* (*IJCP*) which looked at twenty-one studies carried out over 27 years.[50] In total, about 37,000 women had been involved.

They concluded that aspirin could reduce the risk of breast cancer by 20 per cent. They also suggested that other NSAIDs could offer protection as well. They were unable to give recommendations on dosage or duration of treatment needed.

They did not feel, however, that on the strength of their findings they could recommend that women should start taking NSAIDs to prevent breast cancer in view of the risk of side effects. More research was needed.

### Improved survival?

In 2010, a paper was published in the *Journal of Clinical Oncology* by a team led by Dr Michele Holmes from Harvard in the USA.[51] It looked at the possible use of aspirin in women who had already been diagnosed with breast cancer. This was the first study to look at aspirin's use as an aid in treatment of breast cancer.

Between 1976 and 2006, 4,164 nurses who had been diagnosed with breast cancer were included. Over the course of the follow-up, 341 patients died from their breast cancer.

The research team reached the following conclusions:

- Aspirin use was associated with a decreased risk for spread, breast cancer death, and death from any cause.
- Depending on weekly dosage of aspirin, patients were able to reduce the risk for spread by metastasis by 43–60 per cent.
- Compared with non-users, aspirin use was associated with a 64–71 per cent reduction in the risk for breast cancer-related death.

However, the researchers were clear in stating that this was an observational study and that it was *not* possible to say that aspirin had improved survival. They suggested that further research would need to be done.

They were also clear in stating that all patients had conventional treatment for their breast cancers and the aspirin was something that was being taken *in addition*. It was not an alternative to treatment. Indeed, the majority were taking the aspirin as a preventive measure against a cardiovascular event.

### CHAPTER SUMMARY

Firstly:

- All women should take advantage of breast screening when they are notified and they should have mammograms.
- If a woman finds a lump in her breast, she should have it checked by a doctor, since swift diagnosis and investigation is most desirable.

In terms of aspirin's role in treating and preventing breast cancer, the research is promising, but insubstantial. Further research is needed.

Early studies suggest that aspirin use could reduce the risk of breast cancer by 20 per cent. In patients with breast cancer, aspirin has been shown to reduce the risk of the cancer spreading by

43–60 per cent, and there was also a 64–71 per cent reduction in the risk of breast cancer-related death. However, there is not yet enough research to suggest that well women should put themselves at risk of having an aspirin-related bleed in order to reduce their risk of breast cancer, as aspirin has *not* been conclusively proven to be a primary preventative agent in breast cancer. Nor is its use as a treatment for breast cancer patients recommended.

However, if a patient's doctor thought that the patient should consider taking aspirin to help prevent cardiovascular events (such as a heart attack or stroke) – a use for aspirin that *has* been conclusively proven to be effective – then provided the patient has no contraindications, some breast cancer protection is quite possible.

# 14
# CANCER OF THE PROSTATE

While breast cancer is the main fear for women, prostate cancer causes almost as much anxiety in men.

> **THE PROSTATE**
>
> The prostate gland is unique to men. It is a gland found at the base of the bladder and in front of the rectum.
>
> The name comes from medieval Latin *prostate*, meaning 'standing before'.

## The prostate gland

The prostate gland has thousands of tiny glands, which produce a fluid that helps to protect and nourish sperm. This fluid forms a large part of the seminal fluid. When a male orgasms, this fluid is expelled from the prostate into the urethra, thereby contributing to the seminal flow ejaculate.

Prostate cancer is usually caused by cancer cells – mainly malignant tumours called adenocarcinoma – forming as little islands in the prostate tissue.

## Some basic statistics

- Prostate cancer is the commonest new cancer in men in the UK – 24 per cent of new cancers.
- Currently, 101 new cases of prostate cancer are diagnosed every day.
- The lifetime risk of developing prostate cancer for men in the UK is 1 in 9.
- The risk of developing prostate cancer is age-related – it is rare below 50 years.
- 75 per cent of those diagnosed are over 65 years old.
- 10,000 deaths per year are due to prostate cancer.

## Prostate cancer

It is estimated from post-mortem analyses that about 50 per cent of all men in their fifties will have some cancer cells in their prostate. This figure rises to 80 per cent at the age of eighty.

For many men, the cancer simply lies dormant and they are unaware of it. This lies in line with the fact that only one in twenty-six men will die from prostate cancer. The younger the age at diagnosis, the more likely is the disease to progress.

- It is still a potentially serious disease, so if men experience problems in passing urine – loss of power, slow stream or delay in initiating a flow of urine – they should seek a medical opinion.
- Benign prostatic hypertrophy is the more likely diagnosis, but testing can exclude or confirm prostate cancer.

> **OLD MAN'S PROBLEM**
>
> In benign prostatic hypertrophy, a non-malignant disease, the prostate gland enlarges until it compresses the urethra, which runs from the bladder down through the penis.
>
> This impinges on the flow of urine and thence produces the characteristic symptoms of loss of power in the stream, delay in initiating a flow and frequency of urination. People refer to it as 'old man's problem'.

# Aspirin and prostate cancer

This is an area of research that is starting to bear fruit, but it is still early days, with the majority of key studies published as recently as 2010. Only further research and time will tell of aspirin's true potential in this field. Overall, however, the signs are promising.

### Risk reduction

A case-control study published in the *American Journal of Epidemiology* in 2010[52] by a group working in several centres in the USA looked at the effect of aspirin and other NSAIDs on the risk of developing prostate cancer.

- 1,001 patients with diagnosed prostate cancer were compared with 942 cancer-free control patients.
- Men who were currently taking aspirin were 21 per cent less likely than those who never used aspirin to have developed prostate cancer.

- Men who had taken aspirin for 5 years or more were 24 per cent less likely than those who never used aspirin to have developed prostate cancer.
- Men who took a daily low dose of aspirin (81mg) were 29 per cent less likely than those who never used aspirin to have developed prostate cancer.

This research adds to the growing evidence that aspirin seems to have a protective role in reducing the risk of developing prostate cancer.

### Aspirin in diagnosed prostate cancer

In late 2010, a study was presented at the 52nd Annual Meeting of the American Society for Radiation Oncology (ASTRO) in San Diego, USA. The researchers had studied the use of anticoagulants and antiplatelet drugs, including aspirin, on 5,275 men who had been diagnosed with prostate cancer that had not spread beyond the gland, and who had been treated with radiotherapy or surgery.

- 1,982 of the patients were receiving anticoagulants.
- In patients using anticoagulants, the risk of dying from prostate cancer at 10 years reduced from 10 per cent to 4 per cent.
- The risk of metastatic spread was considerably reduced.
- Those with high-risk prostate cancer showed most benefit.
- Aspirin offered greater benefit compared to other anticoagulants.

The researchers concluded that aspirin seems to have a beneficial effect and that the results are promising. Further research is needed.

# CANCER OF THE PROSTATE

## CHAPTER SUMMARY

Aspirin use has been shown to be effective at reducing the risk of prostate cancer.

- In one study, men who took a daily low dose of aspirin were 29 per cent less likely than those who never used aspirin to develop prostate cancer.
- The latest large study on aspirin and cancer[46], cited in chapter 10 on Cancer: A Short Overview (see page 126), indicates that the risk for prostate cancers fell *only after* aspirin had been taken for 15 years.
- After 20 years of aspirin use, the death rate for prostate cancer fell by 10 per cent.
- In one study, aspirin use appeared to reduce considerably the risk of spread of cancer, should prostate cancer be diagnosed.

It is worth noting that prostate problems are most likely to occur at older ages. These ages are also the times when men are more at cardiovascular risk, so if aspirin has already been recommended for improving a patient's cardiovascular risk, the possible reduction in prostate cancer risk would be a bonus.

# ASPIRIN IN DIABETES

Diabetes mellitus is a disorder of carbohydrate metabolism from too little insulin, or from a lack of response to the body's own insulin.

The characteristic feature of diabetes in an undiagnosed or untreated form is excess thirst and increased tendency to pass urine.

## 'The honey-sweet siphon'

Medical writers have been aware of the condition for at least 4,000 years. There is mention of it in the Ebers Papyrus, an Egyptian text from 1,534 BC.

Aretaeus first used the word 'diabetes' in AD 100 to indicate this condition (*dia* meaning 'through' and *betes* meaning 'passing'), likening the passing through of urine to a siphon action.

Dr Thomas Willis, personal physician to King Charles II, and the discoverer of the Circle of Willis (see page 96), stated that diabetic urine was 'wonderfully sweet as if it were imbued with honey or sugar', since tasting patients' urine was an art that most physicians practised in his day. He added the Latin word *mellitus*, meaning 'honey-sweet'.

## The two types of diabetes

1. Type 1 – insulin dependent diabetes mellitus, IDDM. Sometimes referred to as juvenile onset diabetes. It is due to failure to produce insulin. It usually has an early age of onset and requires insulin for life.
2. Type 2 – non-insulin dependent diabetes mellitus, NIDDM. Sometimes referred to as maturity onset diabetes. It is due to lack of response to the body's insulin. Weight and diet control and oral hypoglycaemic drugs may be needed.

## Complications of diabetes

Good diabetes care means good control of blood sugar levels.

There are several possible complications from the condition that may be divided into groups:

* Metabolic – problems with the sugar levels, either from the condition or its treatment
* Vascular – these can be subdivided into:
  1. Macro-vascular – disease of large blood vessels, e.g. coronary arteries (angina and heart attacks), peripheral arteries (intermittent claudication – see page 105), cerebral arteries (strokes)
  2. Micro-vascular – disease of small blood vessels, e.g. diabetic retinopathy (blood vessels in the retinae of the eyes), nephropathy (blood vessels in the kidneys), and neuropathy (blood vessels to the small tissues and the nerves)
* Immune impairment – resulting in more infections
* Cataracts
* Erectile dysfunction and loss of libido

# Do people with diabetes need to take aspirin?

For diabetics under sixteen years of age, the answer is no. Youth has been considered a contraindication against aspirin use since 1979, when it was found that there was a significant link between aspirin and Reye's syndrome (see page 202). Accordingly, aspirin is not recommended to anyone below the age of sixteen years, either with or without diabetes.

For older diabetics, up until 2008 the recommendations were clear: low dose aspirin was recommended for diabetics aged fifty or over, or who'd had diabetes for more than 10 years, and for diabetics receiving treatment for high blood pressure. Unduly high blood pressure had to be treated first.

Yet, as with so many things in science and medicine, things are not always as one would expect. There was no hard evidence that *primary prevention* of a heart attack or stroke was necessary in diabetic patients who were otherwise at low risk.

### The POPADAD Trial

In 2008, a paper was published in the *British Medical Journal* (*BMJ*) about the findings from the Prevention of Progression of Arterial Disease and Diabetes (POPADAD) trial.[53]

The researchers looked at whether aspirin and antioxidants, combined or alone, were superior to placebo when treating diabetic patients who were at risk of developing asymptomatic arterial disease. (That means having disease in the limb, coronary or cerebral arteries, but without it causing any symptoms.) They did a randomized, double-blind, factorial designed placebo-controlled trial.

They found no evidence to support the use of either aspirin or antioxidants in primary prevention of cardiovascular mortality in diabetic patients. In other words, aspirin

> **DIABETES UK RECOMMENDATIONS**
>
> The current recommendations take into account the fact that no obvious difference between diabetics and non-diabetics was found in patients with no evidence of existent cardiovascular disease.
>
> Diabetes UK recommends that:
>
> - Diabetics with no known history of cardiovascular risk should discuss their risk of cardiovascular disease with their medical advisor.
> - People without a history of existent cardiovascular disease may not require aspirin.
> - People with a history of cardiovascular disease should probably be on aspirin, provided they have no contraindications.

neither reduced the risk of diabetic patients contracting arterial disease, nor their risk of dying from it.

## Meta-analyses

Once again, the technique of meta-analysis (combining the findings from good quality independent trials and giving due weight to their results to assess a treatment effect) of several trials has proven useful.

A meta-analysis published in the *BMJ* in 2009 by Georgia de Berardis et al.[54] considered six trials on aspirin in primary prevention of cardiovascular complications in diabetics with no pre-existent cardiovascular disease. They did not find any significant reduction in risk of cardiovascular events for diabetics taking aspirin.

Another meta-analysis published in *Diabetes Care* in 2009

by a group from the Mayo Clinic[55] looked at whether diabetics are more at risk of a primary cardiovascular event than people without diabetes. Two reviewers looked at nine randomized controlled trials, comparing the benefit of aspirin among patients with diabetes compared with patients without diabetes for mortality, heart attack and stroke. No significant difference was found between the two groups. They concluded that the relative benefit of aspirin is similar in the two groups of patients.

**CHAPTER SUMMARY**

- As we saw in chapter 6, aspirin is of uncertain benefit in reducing the risk of having a cardiovascular event (heart attack or stroke) in people who are at low risk. Any benefit would have to be balanced against the risk of having a major bleed. For this reason, diabetics with *no previous history* of cardiovascular disease and who have good control of their diabetes may not need aspirin.
- Vascular complications are more common in diabetics, particularly if diabetes control is not excellent. For this reason, people with poorly controlled diabetes may need to consider taking low dose aspirin, provided there are no contraindications.
- Many people with diabetes, particularly type 1 diabetes, will be under sixteen years of age. Aspirin should not be used in children or adolescents under the age of sixteen because of the risk of Reye's syndrome (see page 202).
- In my opinion, every case has to be considered on its own merits and the person's own GP is excellently placed to advise on the potential benefits or otherwise of low dose aspirin.

# 16

# DEPRESSION

> *In sooth I know not why I am so sad;*
> *It wearies me; you say it wearies you;*
> *But how I caught it, found it, or came by it,*
> *What stuff 'tis made of,*
> *Whereof it is born*
> *I am to learn;*
> *And such a want-wit sadness makes of me,*
> *That I have much ado to know myself.*
>
> The Merchant of Venice (Act I, scene i)
> William Shakespeare

## Some depressing statistics

Depression is extremely common. Sometimes it occurs after an obvious trigger in someone's life, but in many cases it just seems to happen, as if a black shutter is pulled down on the person's feelings.

- Depression affects 2.3 million people in the UK at any time.

- In 30–50 per cent of cases, depression is never diagnosed.
- 60 per cent of people with depression say that they are too embarrassed to seek help from a doctor.
- Depression is potentially life-threatening. About 15 per cent of people with depression commit suicide each year.
- It takes 10 years and £350 million to develop a new antidepressant.
- The global drug market for psychotropic medication is estimated in 2012 at $15 billion.

## A history as long as mankind

Sadness and depression have always plagued mankind and have always been a mystery.

### Melancholia

The ancient Greeks believed that lowness of the mood was a manifestation of an imbalance in the body fluids that they called humors. They called it *melancholia* from the Greek *melas*, meaning 'black' and *chole*, meaning 'bile'. According to their Doctrine of Humors, an excess of black bile was the cause. This was the standard medical theory until the Renaissance.

### The master of emotions

William Shakespeare (1564–1616) was a master at describing virtually every emotion that people could experience. His descriptions are classic and would not look out of place in any modern-day psychiatric textbook.

He opens the play *The Merchant of Venice* (1596–98) with the little speech that I have quoted above by a character called Antonio, who is suffering from a depression that he cannot understand. This is exactly what most people with depression experience: confusion about why they should be feeling so low. They may have everything going for them in their lives, yet they still feel emotionally flat and depressed.

## The Anatomy of Melancholy

In 1621, Robert Burton, an Oxford don, published *The Anatomy of Melancholy*, a six-volume work, which was essentially the first major textbook on the subject of depression. It covered the subject from the viewpoints of astrology, medicine, philosophy and proto-psychology.

In it, he produced a model of consciousness, which, although flawed, gave a framework with which people could work. Its influence continued for at least two centuries and it remains a fascinating classic of Renaissance literature.

Burton described 'causeless melancholia', the type that just descends upon a sufferer for no reason, much as Shakespeare had described it in the character of Antonio. Burton advised that people with melancholia could be helped by getting good sleep, eating healthily, listening to music and talking with good friends.

## Nineteenth century – the beginning of psychiatry

Several doctors attempted to differentiate the different types of melancholia.

- Dr Emil Kraepelin (1856–1926), the father of psychiatry, described *involutional melancholia*, as a state of depression at the menopause – from the Latin *involvere*, the process of enfolding or returning. His belief was that the uterus was shrinking and returning to its immature, infertile state.
- In 1870, Dr Henry Maudsley wrote *Body and Mind: An Inquiry into their Connection and Mutual Influence*, one of the first texts to try to understand the nature of the mind in

sickness and in health. In 1926, he founded the world-famous Maudsley Hospital in London for the care of people with mental and emotional problems.

## Twentieth century – different directions

The twentieth century saw the development of three streams of practice in psychiatry.

1. Psychotherapy – following the work of:
   - Sigmund Freud and psychoanalysis
   - Carl Jung and Jungian analysis
   - Alfred Adler and his Individual Psychology

   Essentially, the psychotherapy approach is based upon understanding the thought processes and mental mechanisms that have brought about a certain mental state or condition. The therapies involve resolution of problems by talking.

2. Behaviourist psychology – following the work of Ivan Pavlov and conditioning
   Essentially, the use of various psychological methods to help individuals alter their behaviour and thence improve the way they approach things and how they feel emotionally.

3. Neuro-organic psychiatry
   This subscribes to the view that mental activity is a product of brain function. Conditions like depression therefore may be the result of organic changes within the brain, or of imbalance in various neurotransmitters. Treatments include tranquillizers, antidepressants and electro-convulsive therapy, or ECT.

## Antidepressants

In 1951, the drug isoniazid, which was effective when combined with other drugs in the treatment of tuberculosis, was found to have a mood-elevating effect in depressed patients. It became the first antidepressant.

⬇

In the 1950s and 1960s, the amphetamine group of drugs was widely used in depression.

⬇

In 1957, Roland Kuhn discovered the antidepressant effect of imipramine, the first of the tricyclic group of antidepressants. These drugs seemed to have fewer side effects than the amphetamines.

⬇

In the 1980s, the first selective serotonin re-uptake inhibitor (SSRI) drugs were introduced in Switzerland. They work by stopping the re-absorption of serotonin at nerve ends. This allows serotonin (the happiness chemical) to accumulate in the brain, which lifts mood.

⬇

The SSRI drugs are now the most widely prescribed drugs in the world for depression.

# Biochemical theories of depression

There have been several main theories about the biochemical nature of depression, namely these two:

- Mono-amine hypothesis
- Cytokine hypothesis

### The mono-amine hypothesis

In 1965, Dr Joseph Schildkraut postulated that deficiency of mono-amine neurotransmitters, or natural messenger chemicals in the brain, had a significant role in depression. The mono-amine hypothesis seems to account for the way in which most of the antidepressants that are commonly prescribed work.

It has its critics, however, since these antidepressants do not work for everyone who is depressed, and it does not seem to account for the action of some of the newer drugs.

### The cytokine hypothesis

Cytokines are small protein molecules found in the brain, central nervous system and the immune system. They are involved in cell-signalling, meaning that they transmit information between cells and may be involved in instructing them to carry out particular functions or actions.

High levels of cytokines are found in people with inflammatory conditions. They are also found in those suffering from depression, which has led researchers to think there may be a link between inflammation and depression. This is of quite marked importance, because it suggests that in some people, depression is a symptom of an inflammatory process that is subtly affecting the brain.

It may also explain why antidepressants do not always work in some people.

## Cytokine and inflammation

It has been well observed that certain groups of people are more likely to become depressed:

- People with auto-immune conditions, like lupus[56]
- People with degenerative conditions, like coronary heart disease and multiple sclerosis[57]
- Elderly people with inflammatory conditions[58]
- Patients receiving cytokine-based immunotherapy treatment

Coupled with these observations are the findings that inflammation and markers of inflammation are linked with major episodes of depression.[59, 60, 61]

This has led to the theory that inflammation itself causes the release of cytokines, which result in depression.

The cytokine hypothesis is a potentially very important concept, since it may offer another way of treating depression (other than SSRI drugs), or of assisting antidepressants to work in people who may have an inflammatory condition present.*

# Could aspirin have an effect on depression?

Starting from the basis that depression seems common in the above groups of people with inflammatory conditions and degenerative conditions that have some inflammatory basis, researchers in Australia hypothesized that two anti-inflammatory agents might have an effect in reducing depression. These two agents were:

---

* However, do see page 204 – some antidepressants interact with aspirin in an unknown way and may increase the risk of a bleed. You should never combine aspirin and antidepressant treatments without first consulting your doctor.

- Aspirin
- Statins – which are used to lower cholesterol

They selected a group of patients who had previously been selected for the Geelong Osteoporosis Study 1994–97 and conducted a nested case-control study.

- 1,494 women had been randomly recruited into the Geelong Study.
- 837 were aged over fifty.
- 386 were assessed after 10 years of follow-up and agreed to take a psychiatric interview.

The research team used a specific interview technique to diagnose episodes of Major Depressive Disorder (MDD) and the age of onset, after the age of fifty. They were specifically interested in the use of statins and aspirin, but also collected information about other NSAIDs, paracetamol, hormones, antidepressants and drugs for diabetes. They performed a retrospective study of a control group with no history of depression, for the same period of time.

The researchers found that 63 patients had a history of depression, but 41 were excluded because they had their depression diagnosed before the age of fifty, which was one of the criteria used for inclusion into this study. This therefore gave them 22 cases to study.

Of the other women in the original group of 383, there were 323 who were eligible to be included as controls, since they had no depression.

## The findings

- The use of statins and aspirin was lower in the women who had a history of depression.
- Only 1 out of 22 women with depression were using statins (around 4.4 per cent), compared with 93 out of 323 women (just under 29 per cent) with no depression.

- Use of aspirin (before the history of depression) was only 1 in 22 women with depression, but 103 in 323 women (almost a third) with no depression.

### The conclusion

The authors wrote about the findings of their study[62] in the *Journal of Psychotherapy and Psychosomatics* in the autumn of 2010. They suggested that there is a **highly significant reduction in the risk of developing major depression if one is taking aspirin** or a statin. They could not explain the difference on the basis of lifestyle or of other drugs.

It seems that the reduction in inflammation seems to be the crux of the matter. This is entirely in keeping with the cytokine hypothesis and with the known facts about aspirin and statins' ability to reduce inflammation.

Although more work needs to be done, it is clear that there is sufficient evidence here to justify further investigation into the cytokine hypothesis and the use of both aspirin and statins in both the treatment and the primary prevention of this highly important condition. But more research needs to be done first.

## How does aspirin help?

It seems plausible that aspirin could be exerting its anti-inflammatory effect by two mechanisms.

1. By its effect on the COX-2 enzyme (see page 49), thereby reducing production of prostaglandins, which in turn reduces the inflammatory response.
2. By inducing the formation of nitric oxide radicals, or NO-radicals, which is another mechanism of aspirin that researchers have discovered. NO-radicals stop white blood cells from sticking together, so may help the body to fight infections.

**CHAPTER SUMMARY**

Some researchers have theorized that depression and inflammation may be linked. As an anti-inflammatory drug, aspirin might therefore be able to prevent depression or reduce its intensity. However, there is not enough evidence at this moment to say that you should take aspirin to reduce the risk of depression. The single study discussed in this chapter is suggestive of a reduction in the risk of developing major depression if one is taking aspirin, but it looked at only a tiny sample of people.

What can be said is that if you had a condition that has an inflammatory component (see page 177 for examples), *and* you were feeling depressed, then aspirin might help. Certainly it would be worth taking this and a past history of depression into account when you sit down with your doctor to discuss whether or not aspirin is something that you should take.

Currently, I believe that the idea of aspirin assisting with depression is merely interesting, yet certainly worthy of further research in well-controlled trials.

# THE SKIN    17

Although aspirin has good anti-inflammatory effects, it has not really been found to be of much use when taken *by mouth* in alleviating skin disorders. In fact, on the contrary, skin rashes such as urticaria (nettle rash or hives) are side effects that are well recognized.

## Aspirin and skin conditions

However, aspirin does have benefits to offer when it comes to the **topical** (i.e. localized and external) use of salicylic acid. Salicyclic acid, as we learned on page 37, is the base form of aspirin, before it has been 'buffered' by the addition of an acetyl group.

Salicylic acid has been used extensively in dermatology (the branch of medicine devoted to the treatment of skin conditions) over the years.

- Salicylic acid is a keratolytic, which means that it softens and removes the outer horny layer of the skin. It does this by breaking down keratin, a protein that forms part of the outer skin. This allows the dead skin to be shed.
- It also has a slight anti-inflammatory effect.
- It is a traditional treatment for psoriasis, a scaling condition that affects the skin.

- It is useful for several other conditions where there is a build-up of the horny layer of the skin – callosities, icthyosis, corns and warts.

## Treatments made with the base form of aspirin

*Lassar's paste* – this is a paste made of zinc oxide and salicylic acid paste. Zinc has astringent properties, meaning it helps the tissues to contract so it also helps to shed loose dead skin.

It is a long-standing treatment for psoriasis and other conditions where the skin outer layers build up.

*Salicylic acid and lactic acid* – this is commonly used as a topical treatment for warts and verruccas, callosities and corns. The presence of the lactic acid makes the salicylic acid more available.

*Salicylic acid, dithranol and coal tar ointment* – this is a mixture of topical preparations that is useful in psoriasis. The dithranol slows down the process of skin cell production, and the salicylic acid acts as a keratolytic to soften and shed the dead skin.

*Salicylic acid and podophyllum resin* – this is used in the treatment of warts. The podophyllum is deadly to the wart-virus-infected cells and the salicylic acid helps to shed them through its keratolytic action.

*Salicylic acid and betamethasone* – this is a mixture of salicylic acid and a steroid, used in types of eczema, especially if there is thickened skin. The steroid betamethasone will help to reduce infection and the salicylic acid will help to shed the dead skin.

*Salicylic acid and sulphur shampoo* – this is used for dandruff and itchy scalp conditions.

# When not to use aspirin

None of these preparations should be used if:

- The patient is allergic to aspirin.
- The skin is broken.
- The skin is inflamed, possibly infected.
- There is peripheral arterial disease (see page 104 – essentially, a hardening of the arteries which affects the limbs).
- There is a mole or undiagnosed skin lesion present.

### HOME REMEDIES

This chapter has examined uses of salicylic acid in medicine. However, there are various home remedies for which people use aspirin as well, which we shall consider in chapter 18 on Unusual Uses of Aspirin.

### CHAPTER SUMMARY

When used in its base form of salicylic acid as a topical, external treatment, aspirin can help with a range of skin conditions, including psoriasis, callosities, icthyosis, corns, warts, verruccas, dandruff and itchy scalp conditions, as well as some types of eczema. The salicylic acid can be combined with other substances to produce pastes and creams that can be put to good medical use.

As usual, anyone with an allergy to aspirin or any other contraindications should not use aspirin, even for this external use.

# UNUSUAL USES OF ASPIRIN 18

We have so far examined the many amazing uses of aspirin medically, including its potential for substantially lowering illness and mortality from a number of conditions. It is exciting to see this, since aspirin does truly seem to have significant potential in many areas of medicine.

Yet it was not always like that. For many years, the drug was considered to be a joke, both within the medical profession and outside it.

## Plum out of it!

The following little snippet says it all.

> A doctor and a plumber were both freemasons and belonged to the same Masonic Lodge. One Sunday night in the early hours, the doctor woke up to find that his toilet was blocked, so he phoned his fellow freemason, the plumber.
>
> The plumber was not pleased. 'But I don't work at night!' he snapped down the phone. 'Can't it wait until tomorrow?'
>
> The doctor was even less pleased at this response. 'Well, I don't like working at nights either, but if I am called out, I always attend.'

'Right!' the plumber replied. 'I'll call round and see what I can do.'

Half an hour later, he arrived and followed the doctor upstairs to look at the toilet.

'Ah, I see,' he said, taking two aspirins from his pocket and throwing them into the bowl. 'There, that should do it. Now, if it is no better in the morning, give me another call and I'll have another look.'

The popular idea was that when doctors wanted to fob someone off, they gave a couple of aspirin.

How things have changed!

## Non-medical uses of aspirin

In medical research, we differentiate experiments into *in vitro* tests, meaning test tube or laboratory tests, from *in vivo* tests, or experiments carried out with living systems.

In the book so far, we have mainly been looking at the effects of aspirin *in vivo*, in the body. The interesting thing is that through *in vitro* tests, aspirin seems to have found several uses that are outside its normal medical use.

## Plant science

The history of aspirin began with plants. This clearly begs the question of why plants should contain salicylates (essentially plant hormones – see page 33), which has generated a huge amount of research in botany and plant science.

Rather than giving an exposition about botany, however, we shall look at some of the unusual uses for which aspirin has been advocated, and then we will look at the scientific basis for them.

## Aspirin keeps cut flowers fresh

Well, it does not quite do that, but it does help them last longer.

Florists regularly use aspirin in the water they keep cut flowers in. It has also been a piece of household lore that dropping an aspirin into a vase will help flowers to keep their blossom for longer than usual.

*Explanation*

Cut flowers are wounded and dying plants. The act of cutting them from the mother plant starts the process known in botany as *senescence*. This is the name given to the ageing process that will result in death. It is under the control of plant hormones.

There are two principal plant hormones involved in this process:

- Ethylene (the gas that you detect when plants and fruits become overripe and die)
- Abscisic acid

Salicylic acid (the base form of aspirin) blocks ethylene and thereby slows down the senescence process, resulting in the flowers lasting longer. Salicylic acid also seems to inhibit the action of abscisic acid.

*Method*

One soluble aspirin to a vase of water.

## Aspirin helps plants to yield more

Because of the common practice of using aspirin to help cut flowers last longer, some gardeners empirically added aspirin to water that is sprayed on various fruits.

Research begun at the University of Rhode Island in 2005 shows that some plants literally yield more when sprayed with aspirin in water. Other universities are following up this research.

## SPECTACULAR RESULTS

Martha McBurney, the master gardener in charge of the vegetable garden at the University of Rhode Island, apparently read an article in a gardening journal which said that aspirin was an activator of 'systemic acquired resistance'. She started spraying tomato and other fruits every three weeks. The results at the end of the season were spectacular. Plants were large, green and insect-free.

Seeds that had been sprayed with aspirin water directly after sowing resulted in 100 per cent germination, compared with spotty germination of others that had been merely watered.

*Explanation*

This is all to do with plant hormones. Salicylates are now considered as plant hormones. Their function is to:

- Regulate plant growth
- Induce disease resistance
- Prolong flower life
- Inhibit ethylene release
- Counteract abscisic acid
- Be an anti-transpirant – i.e. induce the leaves to close their stomata so they do not lose water

*Method*

Care has to be taken. Research shows that plants vary in their ability to tolerate salicylic acid application. Too much aspirin and too frequent watering will cause plants to burn.

The dosage recommended after the University of Rhode

Island experiment is one 300mg aspirin per two gallons of water. The aspirin should be crushed into a fine powder and should be a generic tablet containing only acetylsalicylic acid. The addition of two tablespoons of yucca extract is advised to help the solution stay on the plant leaves and will tend to prevent beading.

### Aspirin as an anti-fungal agent in gardening

Gardeners have also found that aspirin-treated water will reduce the risk of moulds or insect or other pest attacks when soil is watered at the time of planting.

*Explanation*
Salicylic acid is a very mild anti-bacterial and anti-fungal agent in its own right.

The aspirin will be absorbed by the root system or by the seed and will induce the systemic acquired resistance in the plant.

*Method*
One aspirin, or 300mg, per two gallons of water.

## More non-medical uses of aspirin

> **WARNING: ASPIRIN OR NSAID ALLERGIES ARE A TABOO FOR THE FOLLOWING USES**
>
> Some people are genuinely allergic to aspirin. If this is suspected, then they should not take aspirin by mouth, nor should they use aspirin in any of the following applications to the body.

## Aspirin reduces green hair phenomenon

For blonde or light-haired swimmers, trips to the swimming pool can be a source of anxiety because a greenish tinge to the hair can be the result of repeated or prolonged exposure to public swimming pool water. Using water with aspirin dissolved in it will reduce the green effect.

*Explanation*
People mistakenly believe that chlorine in the water is the cause. In fact, the green tinge is usually due to exposure to the salts of dissolved hard metal such as copper, iron and manganese in the water. These may be present as algaecides (anti-algae agents) or in ionic form as a result of ionization. The dissolved metals attach to the hair, and the chlorine content of the water then oxidizes them to produce the green tinge. Aspirin is a mild acid and it will remove the oxidized metals from the hairs.

*Method of application*
This is not to be taken by mouth.

Crush two generic aspirin tablets in a litre of water and use this to wash your hair. Let it soak for a couple of minutes, then rinse off thoroughly.

## Aspirin can help to remove perspiration stains

Perspiration has a similar composition to urine, except it has about $1/130^{th}$ of the amount of urea. It does not smell the same, but if someone tends to perspire a lot, the perspiration will impregnate the clothing and may well leave a yellowish stain when it dries. This is most usually seen on caps and hat-bands, inside neck collars and under the arms in T-shirts and shirts.

If an anti-perspirant is used, then this can compound matters. Most anti-perspirants work by blocking the pores of the skin and thereby the sweat glands. The chemical that does this is usually aluminium chloride. While it will prevent perspiration for a few hours, it will eventually wear off and some aluminium salts will be deposited in the clothing fibres, undergoing change as they dry and producing a yellowish discolouration.

*Explanation*

The cause of the discolouration is bacterial action of chemicals in the perspiration. There may also be some oxidation of chemicals and reaction with the fibres of the material.

The aspirin works to remove the stains due to its mild acidic effect, and also to the keratolytic effect of acetylsalicylic acid. Keratolytic means that it softens and removes hard particles. It will break surface salts free from the fibres.

*Method of application*

This is to be used topically (in the affected area only). Dissolve two 75mg aspirins in a cup of water and pour onto the stain. Leave to soak into the material for two hours. Then rinse it out and wash as usual.

## Aspirin removes smoking stains from fingers

While aspirin may indeed remove body stains from shirts, I confess to feeling hot under the collar when I discuss this one. Some people smoke so many cigarettes that they produce smoking stains on their fingers. Prevention of these by not smoking is far better than having to apply such a treatment!

These are often thought to be nicotine stains. In fact, they are a mix of nicotine staining and coal tar staining.

*Explanation*

The staining is not just on the surface of the skin but several cells deep. The salicylic acid's keratolytic ability will soften and help those outer layers of cells to shed. The staining will not go until those stained cells are removed.

*Method of application*

This is not to be taken by mouth, but used topically. Dissolve one 75mg aspirin in a cupful of warm water and soak the fingers in this. Rub it all over and keep rubbing for up to five minutes a day. It will take several applications, but it will soon remove the stains. Wash well with water and then apply a moisturizer after each application.

## Aspirin removes tobacco smoke stains from walls

*Explanation*

In this case, the staining is usually on the wall's surface. Here the salicylic acid seems to combine with the coal tar mixture, as it does when making some of the skin creams we considered in the last chapter. Thus a cream is formed that can be wiped or washed away.

*Method of application*

This is to be used topically. A preparation of a 75mg aspirin in a cup of water can be applied with a cloth to areas of wallpaper that have been discoloured by tobacco smoke.

## Aspirin as a treatment for dandruff

Dandruff can be a worrisome condition for many people. The skin cells of the scalp are continually renewing themselves. New cells form in the deeper layers of the skin, and are gradually pushed upwards by new cells forming beneath. As they reach the surface, they become very flat, like tiny plates, which overlap one another. By the time they reach the top, they are dead and are shed unnoticed.

In dandruff, the skin cell turnover is speeded up. In mild cases, tiny flakes of skin are shed to produce a dust-like effect. In more severe cases, there is a clumping of skin cells, producing embarrassing flakes and snowstorms on dark clothes. Often, the scalp feels itchy.

*Explanation*

People with dandruff often have a tiny yeast, called *Pityrosporum ovale*, on their scalp. Everyone has this on their skin, especially on greasy areas such as the scalp, behind the ears and on the back. The dandruff sufferer, however, is liable to have very much more of it.

Whether it is there as a cause or an effect is not known, but diminishing the amount often improves the condition. As aspirin is mildly anti-fungal, it reduces the population of *Pityrosporum ovale*.

Aspirin is also a keratolytic and exfoliator, so it helps to remove partially shed skin cells.

*Method of application*

This is not to be taken by mouth, but applied topically. Dissolve one 75mg aspirin in a little water and mix this with your usual shampoo (but not a selenium-based shampoo – check the ingredients listed on the bottle first). Apply to the hair as normal. Leave for a couple of minutes, then rinse out. Apply two or three times a week.

## Aspirin can shrink a spot or pimple

Aspirin crushed and mixed with enough water to make a paste, then applied to a spot or pimple, may help to shrink it.

*Explanation*

A pimple is a localized area of infection and inflammation. The body is doing its best to overcome the infection and the inflammatory response has been activated (see chapter 5 on Pain, Fever and Inflammation, for an explanation about inflammation, page 60). White cells are accumulating to absorb the bacteria and pus is being formed.

Some of the aspirin applied as a paste will be absorbed into the skin. It blocks the COX-enzyme systems (see page 49) in the tissue, which reduces prostaglandin production and helps to reduce inflammation. It may also stimulate resolvin production (see page 62) to help close down the inflammatory response.

*Method of application*

This is not to be taken by mouth, but applied topically. Crush and dissolve one 75mg aspirin in just enough water (about a teaspoonful) to make a paste. Then apply this to the spot or pimple and leave for two minutes. Then wash off thoroughly with cold water. The process can be repeated after four hours.

This will help to shrink the spot, which will clear up the imperfection faster.

> **Note:** Some people suggest using this aspirin-based paste for acne treatment. You are strongly advised *not* to do this, but instead you should seek help from your GP, since there are effective treatments available.

## Aspirin as a treatment for insect bites

This is another 'home help' treatment, this time for itchy insect bites. A paste made in the same way as above for a pimple treatment, if applied quickly to a midge or mosquito bite, can reduce the swelling, itch and pain from the bite or sting.

*Explanation*

This is exactly the same as for the pimple treatment.

Some people seem to react badly to midge or mosquito bites. It is often assumed that the biting parts or stings were contaminated with bacteria. In fact, most of the reaction is allergic, in that the body reacts to the saliva or the venom in the sting, and it is this which induces the inflammatory response.

*Method of application*

This is not to be taken by mouth, but applied topically. Crush and dissolve one 75mg aspirin in just enough water (about a teaspoonful) to make a paste. Then apply this to the insect bite or sting and leave for two minutes. Then wash off thoroughly with cold water. It can be repeated after four hours.

This will help to relieve the itch and pain.

## Aspirin as a treatment for ingrowing hairs

Women often experience ingrowing hairs after they shave or wax their bikini line. The area around the follicle can become extremely painful and inflamed.

*Explanation*

When hair is shaved, the result will be that its end will be sharp and rather like a sliver. As the hair grows from the base of the hair follicle, the sliver-like hair will bend round and traumatize the inside of its own follicle. This will induce the inflammatory response. This produces swelling around the area and the production of pus.

The aspirin will reduce the inflammatory response by blocking the COX enzyme system and so the production of prostaglandins will be reduced. As the inflammation settles, the swelling will be reduced, and the growing hair with its bent-over 'ingrown' part will be released.

*Method of application*

This is not to be taken by mouth, but applied topically. Crush and dissolve one 75mg aspirin in just enough water (about a teaspoonful) to make a paste. Then apply this to the ingrowing hair and leave for two minutes. Then wash off thoroughly with cold water. It can be repeated after four hours. This will help to relieve the itch and pain.

## Aspirin as a treatment for callus or callosity removal

Hard calluses on the balls of the feet or the heels can be softened with aspirin, so that they can be gently pumiced away.

*Explanation*

A callus is a build-up of thickened skin that has been the result of repeated pressure and friction on the part. Aspirin is a keratolytic and exfoliator, so it will help to soften the dead skin, making it easier to remove.

*Method of application*

This is not to be taken by mouth, but applied topically

Crush and dissolve four 75mg aspirin in just enough water (about a tablespoonful) to make a paste. Soak this onto a flannel and apply to the callus. Leave this on for about ten minutes, then remove and wash away and dry. Then gently pumice the area. Do this on a daily basis for a week.

# 19 ASPIRIN: SIDE EFFECTS AND PRECAUTIONS

Throughout this book, we have alluded to possible side effects that may preclude the taking of aspirin for some people. This is very important, because aspirin is simply not a drug that everyone can take.

In chapter 4 on How Aspirin Works, we looked at the scientific mechanisms that bring about both its benefits and many of its side effects. It is because it has both that we know that it is a very powerful drug, far more powerful and useful than could ever have been imagined when Felix Hoffman first produced it back in 1897.

**The side effects are very important. Your doctor will cover these with you, but you should be aware of the following topics.**

## Gastrointestinal side effects

The commonest side effects reported are:

- Irritation of the stomach and intestines
- Indigestion and heartburn
- Nausea

To put this in proportion, about 6 per cent of people will experience some form of indigestion.

> **WARNING**
>
> Anyone with a history of stomach ulceration should **never** take aspirin.

## The PAIN Study

In 1999, the PAIN study (the Paracetamol, Aspirin and Ibuprofen New tolerability study) was published.[63] This was a large-scale, randomized clinical trial comparing the tolerability of aspirin, ibuprofen and paracetamol for short-term pain relief. Researchers found that of 8,633 patients consulting their GP and being prescribed these three drugs:

- Aspirin was associated with gastric upset in 6.3 per cent of cases.
- Paracetamol was associated with gastric upset in 4.1 per cent of cases.
- Ibuprofen was associated with gastric upset in 2.9 per cent of cases.

## Adverse effects

A Cochrane* meta-analysis of 68 randomized, placebo-controlled trials for post-operative pain was published in 1999. In all, 5,069 patients received either 600–650mg aspirin or a placebo.

---

* The Cochrane Collaboration was established in 1993 and is an independent international network that provides practitioners, consumers and health policy makers with evidence-based research.

- 13 per cent of aspirin-takers reported an adverse effect.
- 11 per cent of placebo-takers reported an adverse effect.

Interestingly, drowsiness was the commonest aspirin adverse effect reported, indicating that it had relieved the pain – so the post-operative drowsiness became more apparent.

### Conclusion

The conclusion of these two studies was that gastric side effects do not seem to be as common as are imagined.

Note: There is evidence that taking aspirin with milk reduces the risk of a gastric upset.

## DANGER SIGNAL – coffee ground vomit or black motions

The most dangerous gastrointestinal side effect of aspirin is that it may cause bleeding in the stomach. If this occurs, then it may make a patient vomit up fresh blood. If the bleeding is not quite so severe, then one may vomit up what looks like coffee grounds. If either of these occur, stop aspirin *immediately* and consult a doctor.

Similarly, if you experience black bowel motions when taking aspirin, stop the drug *at once*. This could be melaena, which means that you are losing blood into the stomach and it is being partially digested. Consult a doctor immediately.

### How common are gastrointestinal bleeds on low dose aspirin?

The answer to this is, they are not common, but they are potentially dangerous.

- There is a twofold increase in the risk of having a major bleed with low dose aspirin as opposed to not having aspirin.

- The overall risk of having a bleed in the gut with low dose aspirin is 1 in 1,000 per year.
- Of these bleeds, only 1 in 20 would be fatal. Thus over a 20-year period, 1 person in 1,000 taking low dose aspirin might have a fatal bleed.
- The risk of having a bleed increases with increasing dosage. At full dosage of up to 1500mg daily, the risk would be four times greater than for low dose aspirin.

## Aspirin hypersensitivity

About 0.5 per cent of the general population will have aspirin hypersensitivity. The two commonest manifestations of hypersensitivity are:

- Bronchospasm, or aspirin-induced asthma.
- Acute hypersensitivity – anaphylactic reaction, urticaria (nettle rash) and angio-oedema. Angio-oedema is intense swelling in the tissues of the skin, often of the lips, throat, nose, tongue and genitals. It can quickly tighten the throat and make breathing difficult. It can occur when one is allergic to certain foods or drugs like aspirin and it should be regarded as a medical emergency.

These side effects actually seem to have two separate mechanisms. Both are serious and potentially dangerous.

### Aspirin-induced asthma

Aspirin can cause bronchospasm and worsen asthma in known asthma sufferers. For this reason, most asthma sufferers are quite correctly advised against using it. The reaction can affect the whole respiratory tract, including the sinuses, the nose and the lungs. The bronchospasm it induces can be extremely severe.

A review was published in the *BMJ* in 2004,[64] which estimated the incidence of worsening bronchospasm in adults with a history of asthma at 21 per cent. That is too high a risk for anyone with asthma. Therefore, **people with a known history of asthma should not take aspirin or other NSAIDs.**

### Acute hypersensitivity reactions

Sudden swelling of the lips, mouth, nose, throat, eyelids and face are all danger symptoms of a serious reaction. Any tightness in the throat or difficulty breathing is a major danger sign. Collapse is possible also. **This is a medical emergency and needs instant treatment.** An appointment to see a doctor later in the day is not good enough; it has to be dealt with urgently.

Less severe reactions are nettle rash and skin irritation.

### Conclusion

- Overall, only about 0.5 per cent of people experience an allergic reaction, but if you develop one, then you should avoid aspirin and other NSAIDs ever after.
- Hypersensitivity to aspirin is lifelong – if it happens once, then aspirin and other NSAIDs should never be taken again.

## Bruising

Easy bruising is a side effect of aspirin that is often written about. It is not clear, however, whether it is as common as people think it might be. In looking at the reporting of bruising by patients taking part in various medical trials of aspirin, bruising has been complained about by 9–43 per cent of controls; that is, in those people who were *not* actually taking aspirin. This compared with 14–53 per cent of those taking aspirin. It is therefore a slight increase, but not a large one.

A study published in 2011[65] found a curious result when they looked at bruising rates in frequent takers of aspirin, non-users of aspirin and occasional users. They found that bruising was commonest in infrequent users, least common in regular aspirin users and mid-way in the non-users.

## Heavier periods

This is another side effect that is occasionally complained of by women taking aspirin. The same study mentioned above found the same curious association as with bruising. However, it does not seem to be a significant problem.

## Haemorrhagic stroke

The risk of having a haemorrhagic stroke is increased when taking aspirin. (Please see chapter 7 on Strokes, page 95, to see the difference between strokes.) It is something that has to be taken into consideration before embarking on aspirin treatment.

A meta-analysis of sixteen trials covering 55,000 patients was published in the *Journal of the American Medical Association* in 1998 and puts this risk in perspective.[66]

- The mean dose of aspirin was 272mg (range 75mg to 1,500mg aspirin per day).
- Average length of the trials was 36 months.
- The rate of haemorrhagic strokes was 0.26 per cent, compared to 0.12 with the controls (non-aspirin takers).

This suggested that for every 715 people treated with aspirin, there would be one extra haemorrhagic stroke. On the other hand, for every 335 people treated with aspirin, there would be one ischaemic stroke prevented.

### Conclusion

- No one with a history of previous haemorrhagic stroke should receive aspirin.
- No one on drugs like anticoagulants, or other drugs which could interact to increase the risk of haemorrhage, should take aspirin.

## Osler-Weber-Rendu disease

Anyone with Osler-Weber-Rendu disease, also known as the condition of hereditary haemorrhagic telangiectasia, should avoid aspirin. This condition is characterized by little knots of blood vessels (telangiectasia) which can bleed spontaneously. They can bleed in the nose to cause nosebleeds, in the skin to cause bruising, or in the stomach and bowel to produce blood loss leading to anaemia.

Aspirin could make such bleeding more likely, so it should be avoided.

## Reye's syndrome

This is a very rare but serious condition that affects the brain and the liver. It is a medical emergency and necessitates urgent treatment to prevent permanent brain and liver damage.

- Almost all cases have occurred in children.
- It occurs when children have been treated with low dose 'junior' aspirin for flu-like illnesses or chickenpox.

## Conclusion

- Aspirin is now no longer given to anyone under the age of sixteen.
- Aspirin should not be given to women who are breast-feeding.

## Aspirin and surgery

It is usual practice to advise people to stop taking aspirin before a planned surgical procedure for 5–9 days before the operation, because there is a tendency to bleed more. However, patients at high risk of a thrombotic event (i.e. a heart attack or stroke) will swiftly lose their protection and the risk of an event may be more than the risk of bleeding with the surgery.

It is important to discuss with your doctor and your surgeon whether daily aspirin should be stopped before surgery and for how long beforehand.

## Drug and herbal interactions

It is important that you always consult with your doctor when you decide to take any medication other than the ones that are prescribed. You should certainly check that it is OK to take any supplements or herbs if you are taking aspirin.

### Drugs that may interact with aspirin

The generic drug terms used here may not be familiar to all readers, unless you have been prescribed them in the past. However, it's a useful list to consult when considering embarking on aspirin treatment, and will enable you to watch out for possible clashes should you find yourself on multiple drug courses at any one time.

- Alcohol – potentially aspirin and alcohol can in combination produce a gastrointestinal bleed. This is not likely as long as the recommended limits are observed. Any more than that and it could be a hazard.
- Anticoagulants – aspirin may increase the risk of haemorrhage.
- Beta-blockers – aspirin may reduce their effect.
- Carbonic anhydrase inhibitors – such as acetazolamide, used in the treatment of glaucoma. It reduces the effect of aspirin.
- Insulin and oral hypoglycaemics – aspirin may interact and provoke hypoglycaemia (when blood sugar levels fall below the normal level).
- Methotrexate – aspirin may produce side effects with it.
- Valproic acid – aspirin may produce side effects with it.
- Angiotensin-converting enzyme (ACE) inhibitors – an anti-hypertensive, whose effect may be reduced by aspirin.
- Diuretics – their effect may be reduced by aspirin.
- Some antidepressants – they have an uncertain effect on aspirin and may increase the risk of a bleed.
- Other NSAIDs – may increase the risk of a bleed.

## Herbal preparations and supplements that may interact with aspirin

- Danshen
- Dong quai
- Evening primrose oil
- Ginkgo
- Omega-3 fatty acids (fish oil)
- Willow bark

## ASPIRIN: SIDE EFFECTS AND PRECAUTIONS

### CHAPTER SUMMARY

While most people can take aspirin, it is a powerful drug and does have side effects for some patients. If you ever experience side effects with aspirin, it can mean that you should not take it in the future. This is why it's so important to discuss your medical history with your doctor before starting to take aspirin. In some cases, aspirin can be fatal. Do not take the risk.

Side effects include:

- Gastrointestinal problems, from indigestion to stomach ulceration: 6 per cent of aspirin users report gastric irritation
- Gastrointestinal bleeding, affecting 1 in 1,000 people taking low dose aspirin per year, which can lead to the following medical emergencies (and can be fatal to 1 in 20 of those affected):
  o Vomiting of fresh blood
  o Coffee ground vomiting
  o Black bowel motions
- An increased risk of bleeding, including haemorrhagic stroke (a risk for 1 in 700 patients taking low dose aspirin per year)
- An allergy to aspirin, which may present itself as nettle rash or swelling of the lips or, more seriously, provoke an anaphylactic shock: affects 0.5 per cent of people
- Aspirin-induced asthma attacks
- A slight increase in risk of bruising

You should *never* take aspirin if you:

- Have a history of stomach ulceration
- Have a history of asthma
- Have had a haemorrhagic stroke
- Have any blood disorder or inherited condition such as Osler-Weber-Rendu disease, which could predispose you to bleeding

- Have had an allergic reaction to aspirin at any time in your life
- Have a history of salicylate allergy
- Are under sixteen years old
- Are breastfeeding
- Are pregnant (unless prescribed aspirin by a doctor for a specific illness)
- Are trying to conceive
- Are on drugs like anticoagulants, or other drugs which could interact with aspirin to increase the risk of a bleed

# CONCLUSION
# ASPIRIN REFLECTIONS

Writing this book on aspirin has inevitably made me look back at some of the changes I have seen in medical practice over the years. Forgive me now for drifting into a little anecdotage.

Back in the early 1970s, doctors and medical students all wore white coats. As a medical student, my pockets bulged with my stethoscope, patella hammer and the various reference books that you had to carry about. There was a diary to jot down all the investigations, there was a book with all the latest drugs and doses, and there was a book that everyone seemed to have with instructions about what to do in every medical emergency situation. This last book had been written just before aspirin's beneficial effects were published, so there was no mention of it. Instead, after a heart attack, we were advised to treat pain with morphine or heroin (diamorphine), and to use heparin, an anticoagulant, to prevent DVT.

When I qualified and worked as a house physician in cardiology in the mid-1970s, it was my job to admit patients to the coronary care unit. I took their medical history, examined them, took blood for the various tests and started their treatment. Aspirin had just hit the medical headlines and it was given routinely to everyone, provided they had no history of stomach ulceration or of allergy. I dutifully prescribed it, but I have to say that my consultant was not sure whether it actually did very much. Even in medical circles, it was not fully accepted and many doctors were concerned about the risk of a gastrointestinal bleed and were reluctant to use it. Most people had more faith in the intravenous drips, injections and the high-tech paraphernalia of the coronary care unit itself.

Years later, when I was in practice as a GP, I revelled in being on call and having to dash out in the middle of the night to do an emergency home visit. This was the time before paramedics, when the GP was the first person to be called out to attend on medical emergencies. Aspirin was by then well-established as an immediate treatment after a heart attack and, like all GPs, I kept a small bottle in my black bag. Yet even so, it was the injection of a painkiller or of a drug that eased their breathing that people were most grateful for.

Now that aspirin's benefits are being demonstrated in various clinical trials, two things stand out for me. Firstly, it is curious that heroin and aspirin, both drugs developed by Felix Hoffman at the end of the nineteenth century, have had such a major part to play in the treatment of heart attacks. Secondly, it has made me realize how many lives were probably saved by those little aspirin tablets rather than by all of the expensive drugs and invasive procedures that are altogether more glamorous.

Thank you, Felix Hoffman, for giving us aspirin.

# GLOSSARY OF TERMS

**acetylsalicylic acid** the chemical name for aspirin

**adenoma** a benign tumour arising from glandular tissue

**adenocarcinoma** a malignant tumour arising from glandular tissue within an organ

**Alzheimer's disease** the commonest form of dementia

**analgesic** painkiller

**anaphylactic reaction** a serious, potentially life-threatening allergic reaction characterized by low blood pressure, shock and difficulty breathing. It is a medical emergency

**angina** extremely tight chest pain caused when the heart is deprived of blood and therefore of oxygen

**angiogenesis** the process in which malignant tumours cause new blood vessels to grow in order to feed themselves

**anticoagulant** a drug to prevent blood coagulation. Heparin and warfarin are examples

**antiplatelet** a drug, such as aspirin, which prevents platelets from sticking together

**anti-pyretic** fever-reducing agent

**artery** blood vessel that carries oxygenated blood away from the heart, taking it to specific organs

**arteriosclerosis** hardening of the arteries caused by accumulation of atheroma plaque

**atheroma plaque** fatty changes in a blood vessel which form a swelling in the vessel wall

**atrial fibrillation** an irregular beating of the heart caused by loss of the heart's normal pacemaker

**blinded trial** a trial in which the treatment given is not known to people involved. A single-blind trial is when information is held back from the participants, yet the experimenter is fully aware of everything. A double-blind trial is when both the experimenters and the participants are unaware of which treatment is given

**bronchospasm** spasmodic contraction of the smooth muscle in the airways in the lungs, resulting in difficulty breathing

**cancer** umbrella name for a group of conditions in which cells arising from one tissue do not die, but grow and reproduce out of control and out of phase from the rest of the body

**carcinoma** malignancy arising from epithelial cells

**cardiac arrest** the heart stops beating. Unless it is quickly restarted, brain damage or death will swiftly follow

**cardiovascular disease** disease affecting the heart and the blood vessels, which can result in heart attacks, strokes and death

**cerebral artery** *see* artery. A cerebral artery services the brain, providing it with oxygenated blood

**cerebral embolism** when an embolus from the heart (usually from atrial fibrillation) lodges in a brain blood vessel to cause a stroke

**cerebral thrombosis** blood clot forming in a brain blood vessel

**cerebrovascular accident** also known as a CVA, the name for a stroke

**controlled trial** when two groups are identically matched. The treatment group receive a treatment and the other does not

**cohort** sample

**colonoscopy** a fibrescopic examination of the colon

**coronary artery** *see* artery. A coronary artery services the heart muscle itself, providing it with oxygenated blood

**coronary thrombosis** blood clot forming in a coronary (heart) artery

**COX enzymes** cyclo-oxygenase enzymes, involved in producing prostaglandins and thromboxane. Aspirin blocks their effect

**double-blind trial** *see* blinded trial

## GLOSSARY OF TERMS

**DVT** deep-vein thrombosis (DVT) is the name for a thrombus or clot that forms in one of these veins of the lower limb

**embolism** the damage that occurs when an embolus lodges in a blood vessel. *See also* cerebral embolism, pulmonary embolism

**embolus** a fragment of a clot carried in the blood

**epithelium** the lining of the blood vessels, made up by a single layer of flat cells called epithelial cells

**factorial trial** a trial designed to evaluate two types of treatment at the same time. The commonest type is a 2 x 2 factorial trial, where you have two active treatments, A and B, and two non-active treatments, placebo A and placebo B. Patients entering the trial are randomized to one of four groups: A + B, A + placebo B, placebo A + B, and placebo A + placebo B. Then A can be compared with all of the patients not receiving B, and B can be compared with all patients not receiving A

**haemorrhagic stroke** a bleed into the brain

**ischaemic stroke** a stroke which happens when a blood clot blocks off an artery in the brain, preventing oxygenated blood from reaching the brain

**Kawasaki disease** an uncommon condition affecting children under five years. It causes rash, fever, lymph gland enlargement. In one in five children who get it, there may be inflammation of the coronary arteries. It is treated in hospital and is a rare example of when aspirin would be given to children

**meta-analysis** a statistical technique for combining and analysing the findings of independent trials

**metastasis** when cancerous cells spread to another part of the body. Also the name for a localization of cells that have spread from a primary tumour

**myocardial infarction** heart attack

**myocardial ischaemia** state in which the heart muscle is deprived of blood and therefore of oxygen

**myocardium** heart muscle

**nested trial** a group of patients with a specified disease are selected from a sample of people. They are then compared with a group of people without the disease, who had also been included within the sample

**NSAIDs** a group of drugs, the Non-Steroidal Anti-Inflammatory Drugs, so named because they reduce inflammation but do not contain steroids. They work by inhibiting the production of prostaglandins. Examples include aspirin and ibuprofen

**placebo** an inactive or 'dummy' treatment

**placebo-controlled trial** when one group is given an active treatment and the other is given an inactive placebo

**platelet** the smallest type of blood cell. It does not contain DNA. Its function is to clump with other platelets to form a clot to plug a bleeding vessel and help heal a wound

**primary prevention** preventing an illness (such as cancer) or event (such as a heart attack) from ever occurring in a patient

**prostaglandin** natural hormones that are involved in many body processes, including pain, tissue injury and inflammation

**pulmonary embolism** when an embolism from a DVT lodges in a lung vessel

**randomized trial** when various treatments are going to be given, patients are randomized to go into one group or another

**resolvins** group of chemical messengers which help to close down the inflammatory response

**salicylates** naturally occurring chemicals related to aspirin. Plants use them as hormones

**salicylic acid** a white crystalline acid used in the manufacture of aspirin and as a topical treatment in various skin conditions

**secondary prevention** preventing a second medical event from happening or an illness from returning in a patient who has previously suffered it

**senile plaques** characteristic pathological changes seen in the brains of people with Alzheimer's disease

**stroke** brain attack as a result of a thrombosis, embolism or haemorrhage. *See also* haemorrhagic stroke, ischaemic stroke

**thromboxane** a chemical messenger made from prostaglandins in platelets, which cause them to clump and stick together

# GLOSSARY OF TERMS

**thromboembolism** blood clot formation in a vessel which can potentially fragment to release a piece of clot (embolus). That broken clot could then lodge in a distant blood vessel as an embolism

**thrombosis** the process of blood clotting

**thrombus** blood clot

**transient ischaemic attack (TIA)** a mini-stroke. *See also* ischaemic stroke

**vascular** anything relating to blood vessels

**vein** blood vessel that returns deoxygenated blood to the heart

# REFERENCES

## Foreword References

1 Elwood, PC, Cochrane, AL, Burr, ML, et al. A randomized controlled trial of acetyl salicylic acid in the secondary prevention of mortality from myocardial infarction. BMJ 1974; 1: 436-440
2 Randomized trial of intravenous streptokinase, oral aspirin, both, or neither among 17,181 cases of suspected acute myocardial infarction: ISIS-2. Lancet 1988; 2: 349-360
3 Antithrombotic Trialists' Collaboration. Collaborative meta-analysis of randomized trials of antiplatelet therapy for prevention of death, myocardial infarction, and stroke in high risk patients. BMJ 2002; 324: 71-86
4 Antithrombotic Trialists' Collaboration. Aspirin in the primary and secondary prevention of vascular disease: collaborative meta-analysis of individual participant data from randomized trials. Lancet 2009; 373: 1849-60
5 Rothwell, PM, Fowkes, FGR, Belch, JFF, Ogawa, H, Warlow, CP, Meade, TW. Effect of daily aspirin on long-term risk of death due to cancer: analysis of individual patient data from randomized trials. Lancet 2011; 377: 31-41

## Main Text References

1 Nunn, JF. Ancient Egyptian Medicine, British Museum Press, 1996
2 For information about The Aspirin in Reducing Events in the Elderly (ASPREE) study, see www.ASPREE.org
3 Vane, JR. Inhibition of prostaglandin synthesis as a mechanism of action for aspirin-like drugs. Nature 1971; 231: 232-235

# REFERENCES

4   Smith J, Willis A. Aspirin selectively inhibits prostaglandin production in human platelets. Nature 1971; 231: 235-237
5   Eccles, R, Loose, I, Jawad, M, Nyman, L. Effects of acetylsalicylic acid on sore throat pain and other pain symptoms associated with acute upper respiratory tract infection. Pain Medicines 2003; 4: 118-24
6   Rasmussen, BK. Epidemiology of headache. Cephalalgia 1995; 15: 45-68
7   Steiner, TJ, Lange, R, Voelker, M. Aspirin in episodic tension-type headache: placebo-controlled dose ranging comparison with paracetamol. Cephalalgia 2003; 23: 59-66
8   Lipton, RB, Goldstein, J, Baggish, JS, et al. Aspirin is efficacious for the treatment of migraine. Headache 2005; 45: 283-92
9   Elwood, PC, Cochrane, AL, Burr, ML, et al. A randomized controlled trial of acetyl salicylic acid in the secondary prevention of mortality from myocardial infarction. BMJ 1974; 1: 436-440
10  Randomized trial of intravenous streptokinase, oral aspirin, both, or neither among 17,181 cases of suspected acute myocardial infarction: ISIS-2. Lancet 1988; 2: 349-360
11  Antiplatelet Trialists' Collaboration. Secondary prevention of vascular disease by prolonged antiplatelet treatment. BMJ (Clin Res Ed) 1988; 296: 320-331
12  Antiplatelet Trialists' Collaboration. Collaborative overview of randomized trials of antiplatelet therapy. I: Prevention of death, myocardial infarction, and stroke by prolonged antiplatelet therapy in various categories of patient. BMJ 1994; 308: 81-106
13  Antithrombotic Trialists' Collaboration. Collaborative meta-analysis of randomized trials of antiplatelet therapy for prevention of death, myocardial infarction, and stroke in high risk patients. BMJ 2002; 324: 71-86
14  Final report on the aspirin component of the ongoing Physicians' Health Study. Steering Committee of the Physicians' Health Study Research Group. N Engl J Med 1989; 321(3): 129-35
15  Hansson, L, Zanchetti, A, Carruthers, SG, et al. The HOT Study Group. Effects of intensive blood-pressure lowering and low-dose aspirin in patients with hypertension: principal results of the Hypertension Optimal Treatment (HOT) randomized trial. Lancet 1998; 351: 1755-1762
16  The Medical Research Council's General Practice Research Framework. Thrombosis prevention trial: randomized trial of low-

intensity oral anticoagulation with warfarin and low-dose aspirin in the primary prevention of ischaemic heart disease in men at increased risk. Lancet 1998; 351: 233-41

17 Collaborative Group of the Primary Prevention Project (PPP): Low-dose aspirin and vitamin E in people at cardiovascular risk: a randomized trial in General Practice. Lancet 2001; 357: 89-95

18 Ridker, PM, Cook, NR, Lee, IM, et al. A randomized trial of low-dose aspirin in the primary prevention of cardiovascular disease in women. N Engl J Med 2005; 352: 1293-304

19 Antithrombotic Trialists' Collaboration. Aspirin in the primary and secondary prevention of vascular disease: collaborative meta-analysis of individual participant data from randomized trials. Lancet 2009; 373: 1849-60

20 Fields, WS, Lemak, NA, Frankowski, RF, Hardy, RJ. Controlled trial of aspirin in cerebral ischemia. Stroke 1977; 8: 301-14

21 Farrell, B, Godwin, J, Richards, S, Warlow, C. The United Kingdom transient ischaemic attack (UK-TIA) aspirin trial: final results. J Neurol Neurosurg Psychiatry 1991; 54: 1044-54

22 International Stroke Trial Collaborative Group. The International Stroke Trial (IST): a randomized trial of aspirin, subcutaneous heparin, both, or neither among 19,435 patients with acute ischaemic stroke. Lancet 1997; 349: 1569-81

23 Chinese Acute Stroke Trial Collaborative Group. CAST: randomized placebo-controlled trial of early aspirin use in 20,000 patients with acute ischaemic stroke. Lancet 1997; 349: 1641-9

24 Mant, J, Hobbs, R, Fletcher, K, Roalfe, A, Fitzmaurice, D, Lip, GYH, Murray, E on behalf of the BAFTA investigators the Midland Research Practices Network (MidReC). Warfarin versus aspirin for stroke prevention in an elderly community population with atrial fibrillation (the Birmingham Atrial Fibrillation Treatment of the Aged Study, BAFTA): a randomized controlled trial. Lancet 2007; 370: 493-503

25 CAPRIE Steering Committee. A randomized, blinded trial of clopidogrel versus aspirin in patients at risk of ischaemic events (CAPRIE). Lancet 1996; 348: 1329-39

26 Nielsen, GL, Sørensen, HT, Larsen, H, Pedersen, L. Risk of adverse birth outcome and miscarriage in pregnant users of non-steroidal anti-inflammatory drugs: population based observational study and case-control study. BMJ 2001; 322: 266-270

27 CLASP: a randomized trial of low-dose aspirin for the prevention

and treatment of pre-eclampsia among 9,364 pregnant women. Lancet 1994; 343: 619-629
28 Askie, LM, Duley, L, Henderson-Smart, DJ, Stewart, LA, on behalf of the PARIS Collaborative Group. Antiplatelet agents for prevention of pre-eclampsia: a meta-analysis of individual patient data. Lancet 2007; 369: 1791-1798
29 Harris, WH, Salzman, EW, Athanasoulis, CA, Waltman, AC and DeSanctis, RW. Aspirin prophylaxis of venous thromboembolism after total hip replacement. N Engl J Med 1977; 297: 1246-1249
30 Department of Health. Report of the independent expert working group on the prevention of venous thromboembolism in hospitalized patients, 2007
31 National Clinical Guideline Centre. Venous thromboembolism: reducing the risk of venous thromboembolism (deep-vein thrombosis and pulmonary embolism) in patients admitted to hospital, 2010
32 Loke, YK, Derry, S. Air travel and venous thrombosis: how much help might aspirin be? Medscape General Medicine 2002; 4: 3
33 McGeer, PL, Schulzer, M, McGeer, EG. Arthritis and anti-inflammatory agents as possible protective factors for Alzheimer's disease: a review of 17 epidemiological studies. Neurology 1996; 47: 425-432
34 Zandi, PP, Anthony, JC, Hayden, KM, Mehta, K, Mayer, L, Breitner, JCS, for the Cache County Study Investigators. Reduced incidence of AD with NSAID but not H2 receptor antagonists. Neurology 2002; 59: 880-6
35 Kang, JH, Cook, N, Manson, J, Buring, JE, Grodstein, F. Low dose aspirin and cognitive function in the women's health study cognitive cohort. BMJ 2007; 334: 987-990
36 Vlad, SC, Miller, DR, Kowall, NW, Felson, DT. Protective effects of NSAIDs on the development of Alzheimer disease. Neurology 2008; 70: 1672-1677
37 Szekely, CA, Green, RC, Breitner, JCS, et al. No advantage of A 42-lowering NSAIDs for prevention of Alzheimer dementia in six pooled cohort studies. Neurology 2008; 70: 2291-2298
38 Doll, R, Peto, R. The causes of cancer: quantitative estimates of avoidable risks of cancer in the United States today. Oxford University Press 1981
39 Dannenberg, AJ, DuBois, RN (eds). Progress in experimental

tumour research vol 37: COX-2 A new target for cancer prevention and treatment. Karger 2003 (abstr)
40 Tsujii, M, Kawano, S, Tsuji, S, Sawaoka, H, Hori, M, DuBois, RN. Cyclo-oxygenase regulates angiogenesis induced by colon cancer cells. Cell 1998; 93: 705-716
41 Thun, MJ, Henley, SJ, Patrono, C. Non-Steroidal Anti-Inflammatory Drugs as anti-cancer agents: mechanistic, pharmacologic, and clinical issues. J National Cancer Institute 2002; 94; 252-66
42 Rothwell, PM, Wilson, M, Elwin, CE, Norrving, B, Algra, A, Warlow, CP, Meade, TW. Long-term effect of aspirin on colorectal cancer incidence and mortality: 20-year follow-up of five randomized trials. Lancet 2010; 376: 1741-1750
43 Rothwell, PM, Fowkes, FGR, Belch, JFF, Ogawa, H, Warlow, CP, Meade, TW. Effect of daily aspirin on long-term risk of death due to cancer: analysis of individual patient data from randomized trials. Lancet 2011; 377: 31-41
44 Baron, JA, Cole, BF, Sandler, RS, Haile, RW, Ahnen, D, Bresalier, R, McKeown-Eyssen, G, Summers, RW, Rothstein, R, Burke, CA, et al. A randomized trial of aspirin to prevent colorectal adenomas. N Eng J Med 2003; 348: 891-899
45 Sandler, RS, Halabi, S, Baron, JA, Budinger, S, Paskett, E, Keresztes, R, Petrelli, N, Schilsky, R. A randomized trial of aspirin to prevent colorectal adenomas in patients with previous colorectal cancer. N Eng J Med 2003; 348: 883-890
46 Flossmann, E, Rothwell, PM, for the British Doctors Aspirin Trial and the UK-TIA Aspirin Trial. Effect of aspirin on long-term risk of colorectal cancer: consistent evidence from randomized and observational studies. Lancet 2007; 369: 1603-13
47 Rothwell, PM, Wilson, M, Elwin, C-E, Norrving, B, Algra, A, Warlow, CP, Meade, TW. Long-term effect of aspirin on colorectal cancer incidence and mortality: 20-year follow-up of five randomized trials. Lancet 2010; 376: 1741-750
48 Akhmedkhanov, A, Toniolo, P, Zeleniuch-Jacquotte, A, Koenig, KL, Shore, RE. Aspirin and lung cancer in women. British Journal of Cancer 2002; 87: 49-53
49 Moysich, KB, Menezes, RJ, Ronsani, A, Swede, H, Reid, ME, Cummings, KM, Falkner, KL, Loewen, GM, Bepler, G. Regular aspirin use and lung cancer risk. BMC Cancer 2002, 2: 31
50 Agrawal, A, Fentiman, IS. NSAIDs and breast cancer: a possible

prevention and treatment strategy. International Journal of Clinical Practice 2008; 62: 444-449

51 Holmes, MD, Chen, WY, Li, L, Hertzmark, E, Spiegelman, D, Hankinson, SE. Aspirin intake and survival after breast cancer. Journal of Clinical Oncology 2010; 28: 1467-1472

52 Salinas, CA, Kwon, EM, FitzGerald, LM, et al. Use of aspirin and other non-steroidal anti-inflammatory medications in relation to prostate cancer risk. American Journal of Epidemiology (doi: 10.1093/aje/kwq175 First published online: 5 August 2010)

53 Belch, J, MacCuish, A, Campbell, I, et al. The prevention and progression of arterial disease and diabetes (POPADAD) trial: factorial randomized placebo controlled trial of aspirin and antioxidants in patients with diabetes and asymptomatic peripheral arterial disease. BMJ 2008; 337: a1840

54 De Berardis, G, et al. Aspirin for primary prevention of cardiovascular events in people with diabetes: meta-analysis of randomized controlled trials. BMJ 2009; 339: b4531

55 Calvin, AD, Aggarwal, NR, Murad, MH, Shi, Q, Elamin, MB, Geske, JB, Fernandez-Balsells, MM, Albuquerque, FN, Lampropulos, JF, Erwin, PJ, Smith, SA, Montori, VM. Aspirin for the primary prevention of cardiovascular events: a systematic review and meta-analysis comparing patients with and without diabetes. Diabetes Care 2009 (12): 2300-6. Epub 2009

56 Nery, FG, Borba, EF, Viana, VS, Hatch, JP, Soares, JC, Bonfa, E, Neto, FL. Prevalence of depressive and anxiety disorders in systemic lupus erythematosus and their association with antiribosomal P antibodies. Prog Neuropsychopharmacol Biol Psychiatry 2008; 32: 695-700

57 Gold, SM, Irwin, MR. Depression and immunity: inflammation and depressive symptoms in multiple sclerosis. Immunol Allergy Clin North Am 2009; 29: 309-320

58 Milaneschi, Y, Corsi, AM, Penninx, BW, Bandinelli, S, Guralnik, JM, Ferrucci, L. Interleukin-1 receptor antagonist and incident depressive symptoms over 6 years in older persons: The InCHIANTI Study. Biol Psychiatry 2009; 65: 973-978

59 Leonard, BE. Immunological aspects of depressive illness. In Leonard, BE, Miller, K (eds): Stress, the Immune System and Psychiatry. Wiley 1995; 113-136

60 Maes, M, Yirmyia, R, Noraberg, J, Brene, S, Hibbeln, J, Perini, G, Kubera, M, Bob, P, Lerer, B, Maj, M. The inflammatory and

neurodegenerative (IND) hypothesis of depression: leads for future research and new drug developments in depression. Metab Brain Dis 2009; 24: 27-53

61 Kim, YK, Na, KS, Shin, KH, Jung, HY, Choi, SH, Kim, JB. Cytokine imbalance in the pathophysiology of major depressive disorder. Prog Neuropsychopharmacol Biol Psychiatry 2007; 31: 1044-1053

62 Pasco, JA, et al. Clinical implications of the cytokine hypothesis of depression: the association between use of statins and aspirin and the risk of major depression. Journal of Psychotherapy and Psychosomatics 2010; 79: 323-325

63 Moore, N, van Ganse, E, Le Parc, J-M, et al. The PAIN study: Paracetamol, Aspirin and Ibuprofen New tolerability study. A large-scale, randomized clinical trial comparing the tolerability of aspirin, ibuprofen and paracetamol for short-term analgesia. Clin Drug Invest 1999; 18: 89-98

64 Jenkins, C, Costello, J, Hodge, L. Systematic review of prevalence of aspirin-induced asthma and its implications for clinical practice. BMJ 2004; 21; 328 (7437): 434

65 Mauer, AC, Khazanov, NA, Levenkova, N, Tian, S, Barbour, EM, Khalida, C, Tobin, JN, Coller, BS. Impact of sex, age, race, ethnicity and aspirin use on bleeding symptoms in healthy adults. J Thromb Haemost 2011; 9: 100-108

66 He, J, Whelton, PK, Vu, B, Klag, MJ. Aspirin and risk of haemorrhagic stroke: a meta-analysis of randomized controlled trials. J Am Med Assoc 1998; 280: 1930-1935

# INDEX

Locations of major importance are shown in **bold**.

abnormal heart rhythms **75–6**, 77, 78, 101 *see also* heart
acute coronary syndrome (ACS) 77 *see also* heart attacks
adenocarcinomas 17, 143, 148, 156, 161
adenomas 140, 148 *see also* polyps
allergic reactions 18, 30, 82, 188
Alzheimer's disease 17–18, 27, 28, **118–25**
anaphylactic reactions 30, 47, 199, 205
angina 27, 73, **76–7**, 79
anticoagulants: aspirin and 18, 204; elderly people 102; heparin 99; prostate cancer 164; venous thromboembolisms 114; warfarin 43, 89, 101–2
antidepressants 175, 204
anti-inflammatories 25, 26, 57, 121–3, 177–8, 181
arrhythmias *see* abnormal heart rhythms
arteries 52, **70**, **74–5**, 96, **104** *see also* hardening of the arteries
arteriosclerosis *see* hardening of the arteries
arthritis 26, 28, 38, 56, 57, 66
asthma 18, 29, 47, 51, 82, 199–200
atheroma plaque 79
atrial fibrillation **76**, **99–101**; defined 75; dementia and 121; recommendations 15, 28; risk factor 97, **99–101**, treatment 102
autoimmune diseases 108, 167

benign prostatic hypertrophy 162, 163 *see also* prostate cancer
beta-blockers 101, 204
bleeds **52**; anticoagulants 18; aspirin dosage and 150; balancing risk 15, 91, 92; brain 102; breast cancer 17; long usage and 16; minor 23; stomach 30, 51, 102, 198–9; surgery 203
blood 73 *see also* platelets; cells 52, 60, 61, **73**, 80; clots 27, 28, 42, 52, 76 *see also* deep-vein thrombosis; pressure *see* high blood pressure; sugar levels 167; supply **73–5**, 95; tests 81; vessels 47, 50, 61, 65, **72**, 79, 139
bowel cancer *see* colorectal cancer
bowel motions 198
brain: Alzheimer's 120; arteries 52; aspirin's effects 58; bleeds 102; blood supply 95; cancer 17, 29; depression 174; oxygen and 94; risk reduction 90; strokes and 76, 94, 95; tumours 16
breast cancer 126, **157–60**; aspirin and 17, 29, 158–60
breastfeeding 18, 203, 206
breathing difficulties 51, 200
bronchospasm 29, 46, 51, 199–200
bruising 30, 52, 200–201

calluses 195
cancer **126–44** *see also* breast cancer; colorectal cancer; lung cancer; prostate cancer; animal studies

138–9; aspirin 140–4; blocking role in 54; carcinogens 130–1; causes 130–3; cell research 139; classification 133–4; COX-2 138, 139; diet 136; genes 131–2; infections 137; inflammation and 130, 132; metastasis 129, 130, 134, 135, 159, 164; preventative measures 27, 29, 136–7; prostaglandins 138; risk factors 136–8; spreading 128–9; stages 134–5; statistics 126–7; survival rates 44; symptoms 129–30; treatment 135–6; trials 88, 140–3; tumours 127–30, 140; types 16–17; viruses 132–3
cardiac arrests 75 *see also* heart attacks
cardiac rupture 78 *see also* heart attacks
cardiogenic shock 78 *see also* heart attacks
cardiovascular disease 52–4, 67, 68, 169 *see also* heart; heart attacks
cardioversion 101 *see also* heart; heart attacks
cataracts 28, 167
cerebral ischaemia 98
cerebrovascular disease 105, 106
children 18, 30, 42, 168, 203
circulatory system 67, 68, 69, 76, 89
clotting *see* blood: clots
colorectal cancer **145–52**; American research 43; aspirin and 29, 43, 148–52; colon 145–6; distal 147; dosage 150; endoscopies 152; grading 135; improved survival rates 17; polyps 139, 148–9; preventative measures 29; protective factors 147; proximal 16, 147, 151; rectum 146; risk factors 147; running in families 132; statistics 146–7; trials 151
common cold 41, 63–4
coronary arteries **74–5**; blood clots 52; disease 28, 68, 75, 105, 106; infarcts 81; narrowing 76, 79, 80
COX (cyclo-oxygenase) **48–54**; Alzheimer's disease 120, 121; aspirin's effect on 62, 80; cancer 138, 139; depression 179; inflammation 49, 50, 53, 57, 80

dandruff 191–2
deep-vein thrombosis (DVT) 28, **111–16** *see also* thrombosis; risk factors 112
dementia **17–18**, 43, 44, 97, **117–25**
depression 53, **171–80**; antidepressants 175; aspirin and 27, 177–180; biochemical theories 176–7; psychiatric approaches 174; statistics 171–2
diabetes **166–70**; aspirin and 27, 28, 168–70; atrial fibrillation 100; complications 167; heart disease and 79, 167, 169; high blood pressure 168; pregnancy and 108; recommendations 169; strokes and 97, 169; trial 168; types 167
dosage 40, 53–4, 150

elderly people 44, 102, 163
embolisms 28, 95, 102, 121
epithelial cells 72, 79, 80, 139, 142

fever 49, 50, 53, 54, **58–9**
feverish colds 28, 41
forgetfulness 119

gardening 186–8
gastric irritation 21, 22, 23, 25–6, 38, 196–9
gastrointestinal cancers 16
gout 26, 38, **51**
gynaecological cancers 17

haemorrhagic strokes 18, 30, 82, 95, 97, 201–2 *see also* strokes
haemorrhoids 110
hardening of the arteries 72, **79–80**
headaches 28, 49, 57, **64–5**, 96
heart **67–93** *see also* atrial fibrillation; coronary arteries; abnormal rhythms **75–6,** 77, 78, 101; angina 27, 67, 68, 73, **76–7**, 79; aspirin research studies 83–92;

# INDEX

blood supply 73–5; blood vessels 72; cardiac arrest 75; cardiac rupture 78; cardiogenic shock 78; cardiovascular disease 52, 53, 54, 67, 68, 169; cardioversion 101; coronary angiograms 82; diabetes 79, 169; hardening of the arteries 79–80; high blood pressure 78; history of treatment 70–2; irregular heartbeats 97; ischaemic heart disease 89; myocardium 73; oxygen 68–9, 75, 80; pericarditis 28, 78; physiology 68–70; risk factors 78–9; statistics 67–8

heart attacks **14–16, 80–83**; acute coronary syndrome 77; aspirin research studies 83–92; diabetes 167; first 15, 27; immediate treatment after 28; myocardial infarction 77–8; myocardial ischaemia 77, 82; pain from 56; peripheral arterial disease 105; platelets 52, 82; primary heart attack prevention 86–90; problems causing 75; secondary heart attack prevention 27, **83–6**; thrombosis 43, 80; trials 87–90; types of infarct 81

heartburn 23, 29, 196
herbal remedies 203, **204**
hereditary haemorrhagic telangiectasia 18, 202
high blood pressure: diabetes and 168; heart disease and 78; hypertension study 88; in pregnancy 107–9; strokes and 97
high risk patients (heart attack and stroke) 15, **78–9, 97**
hypersensitivity 199
hypertension 88 *see also* high blood pressure

ibuprofen 123, 158, 197
indigestion 29, 196–7, 205
infarcts 81 *see also* heart attacks
inflammation **60–2**; Alzheimer's disease 121, 122; cancer and 130, 132; COX-2 49, 50, 53, 57, 80; depression and 176–7, 179; different mechanisms 54; prostaglandins 43, 47, 57, 58
ingrowing hair 194–5
insect bites 193–4
insulin 166, 167, 204
intermittent claudication 105
intrauterine growth retardation (IUGR) 107–9
irregular heartbeats 97 *see also* atrial fibrillation; heart
ischaemic heart disease (IHD) 89 *see also* heart
ischaemic strokes *see also* strokes; agents against 97; aspirin statistics 202; blood clots 76; low dose aspirin 85; studies 99, 105

Kawasaki disease 28, 211
kidneys 28, 46, 47, 51, 108

Lassar's paste 182
liver disease 97, 110
long-haul flights 114–16
lumbago 41
lung cancer **153–6**; aspirin and 17, 29, 154–6; smoking and 136; statistics 154; types 153

menopause 67
menstrual pain 26, 57, 66, 201
metastatic cancers 129, 130, 134, 135, 159, 164
migraine 28, **65**
Mild Cognitive Impairment (MCI) 119
mini-strokes 15, 87, 98 *see also* strokes
miscarriage 106–7
myocardial infarction (MI) 77–8 *see also* heart attacks
myocardial ischaemia 77, 82 *see also* heart attacks

nausea 29, 196
neuralgia 41, 57
non-haemorrhagic strokes 15, 86
NSAIDs 106–7, 122–4, 138–9, 158, 163

occlusive disease 91, 104
oesophagus 17, 29, 110
Osler-Weber-Rendu disease 18, 202

pacemakers 75–6
pain 49, **55–8**, 60, 77, 78
painkillers 20, 23, 57
palpitations 76
pancreatic cancers 17, 29
paracetamol 25–6, 197
pericarditis 28, 78 see also heart
peripheral arterial disease 100, 104–6
pimples 192–3
platelets see also blood; anti-platelet regimens 85, 97; blood cells 73; blood clots and 27; heart attacks and 52, 82; reducing stickiness 80; strokes 52; thromboxane 52
plaque 75–6
polyps 16, 132, 139, 147–9
portal hypertension 110
post-thrombotic syndrome 111
pre-eclampsia 107–9
pregnancy 18, **106–9**, 112, 116, 206,
preventive uses of aspirin 28–9
prostaglandins **46–52**; Alzheimer's 120, 121; blocking 43, 62; cancer 138; depression 180; inflammation 43, 44, 57, 58; pain and 43, 47, 57–8, 61; reducing 59
prostate cancer **161–5**; aspirin and 16, 17, 29, 163–5; statistics 162
psoriasis 181, 182
pulmonary embolism 28, **111**

rectal cancer see colorectal cancer
Reye's syndrome 30, 42, 168, 170, 202–3
rheumatic fever 26, 28, 38
rheumatism 26, 41, 57

salicylic acid mixtures 182
senile plaques 120
side effects **29–30, 196–206** see also bleeds; stomach: ulceration; asthma 199–200; bruising 200–1; drugs 203–4; gastrointestinal 196–9; haemorrhagic stroke 201–2; heavier periods 201; herbal remedies 203, 204; hypersensitivity 199–200; Osler-Weber-Rendu disease 202; Reye's syndrome 202–3; skin rashes 181; surgery 203; various 22–3
skin cancer 137
skin disorders **181–3**
sore throats 56, **63–4**
stomach: acid 47; bleeds 102; cancer 17; COX-1 49; irritation 51, 53; prostaglandins 46; ulceration 18, 29, 38, 51, 82, 197
strokes **15–16, 94–103**; aspirin research studies 97–102; atrial fibrillation 99–101; COX-2 53; diabetes 167; haemorrhagic 18, 30, 82, 95, 97, 201–2; ischaemic 76, 85, 95, 97, 99; mini-strokes 15, 87, 98; non-fatal 88; non-haemorrhagic 15, 86; oxygen 94; peripheral arterial disease 105; platelets 52; preventative measures 28; risk factors 97; statistics 94; symptoms 95–6; TIAs 98; treatment 96–7; types 27, 95; vascular dementia 121
surgery 135, **203**

temperatures (body) 59; COX-2 49; fever 58; prostaglandins 47, 50; as side effect 30
tension headaches 64–5 see also headaches
therapeutic uses of aspirin 28
thrombosis 28, 53, **80, 88–9**, 95
thyroid 76, 101, 129
TIAs 87, 98

urine 51, 162, 163, 166, 189

varicose veins 110–11
vascular dementia 120–1
veins 70, **110–16**
venous thromboembolism 111–16